Cardiac CT

Zheng-yu Jin • Bin Lu • Yining Wang
Editors

Cardiac CT

Diagnostic Guide and Cases

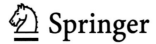

Editors
Zheng-yu Jin
Department of Radiology
Peking Union Medical College Hospital
Chinese Academy of Medical Sciences
and Peking Union Medical College
Beijing
China

Bin Lu
Department of Radiology
Fuwai Hospital
Chinese Academy of Medical Sciences
and Peking Union Medical College
Beijing
China

Yining Wang
Department of Radiology
Peking Union Medical College Hospital
Chinese Academy of Medical Sciences
and Peking Union Medical College
Beijing
China

Associate Editors
Longjiang Zhang
Department of Medical Imaging
Jinling Hospital
Medical School of Nanjing University
Nanjing
Jiangsu
China

Xiaohai Ma
Department of Interventional Diagnosis
and Treatment
Beijing Anzhen Hospital
Capital Medical University
Beijing
China

Dong Li
Radiology Department
Tianjin Medical University General
Hospital
Tianjin
China

Jianxing Qiu
Radiology Department
Peking University First Hospital
Beijing
China

ISBN 978-981-15-5307-3   ISBN 978-981-15-5305-9   (eBook)
https://doi.org/10.1007/978-981-15-5305-9

This Springer imprint is published by the registered company Springer Nature Singapore Pte Ltd.
The registered company address is: 152 Beach Road, #21-01/04 Gateway East, Singapore 189721, Singapore

Preface

Computed tomography (CT) has undergone rapid developments to enable satisfactory performance of cardiac imaging over the last decades. As a result of the improved scanning speed, power boost tubes, and width increased detectors, the latest CT technology enables greater coverage, better spatial and temporal resolution, as well as functional information about cardiac diseases.

The book is case-based and divided into six parts to widely discuss the CT imaging characteristics and applications of coronary artery disease (CAD), non-atherosclerotic coronary artery disease, congenital heart disease, cardiac neoplasms, cardiomyopathy and aortic diseases.

CT angiography imaging was traditionally advantaged in CAD for morphological evaluation of not only coronary arteries stenosis, coronary artery stents and coronary artery bypass grafting, but also non-atherosclerotic coronary artery disease. Further advancement consists of CT dual-energy imaging, CT perfusion imaging and coronary CT angiography derived Fractional flow reserve (CT-FFR), which provide the possibility of functional assessment of myocardial ischemia and myocardial infarction for hemodynamically significant CAD patients. For congenital heart disease and cardiac neoplasms, CT imaging helps in morphological evaluation of the lesion and structure characterization of the whole heart. The diagnostic value of CT examination for cardiomyopathy is still relatively limited for its disadvantage in myocardium evaluation, but recent CT developments enable better evaluation of cardiac functional and myocardium tissue characterization, combined with angiography in one exam. CT angiography has become a most important noninvasive imaging method for the diagnosis, preoperative evaluation and follow-up of aortic diseases.

This contributed book of cardiac CT imaging aims to extensively illustrate case-based cardiac diseases and present the current technical status and applications for readers to systematically understand the performance and interpretation of cardiac CT in clinical practice.

Beijing, China   Zheng-yu Jin
Beijing, China   Bin Lu
Beijing, China   Yining Wang

Contents

Editors and Contributors

Associate Editors

Longjiang Zhang Department of Medical Imaging, Jinling Hospital, Medical School of Nanjing University, Nanjing, Jiangsu, China

Xiaohai Ma Department of Interventional Diagnosis and Treatment, Beijing Anzhen Hospital, Capital Medical University, Beijing, China

Dong Li Radiology Department, Tianjin Medical University General Hospital, Tianjin, China

Jianxing Qiu Radiology Department, Peking University First Hospital, Beijing, China

Contributors

Jian Cao Department of Radiology, Peking Union Medical College Hospital, Chinese Academy of Medical Sciences and Peking Union Medical College, Beijing, China

Qian Chen Department of Medical Imaging, Jinling Hospital, Medical School of Nanjing University, Nanjing, Jiangsu, China

Jingwen Dai Department of Radiology, Peking Union Medical College Hospital, Chinese Academy of Medical Sciences and Peking Union Medical College, Beijing, China

Yan Ding Department of Interventional Diagnosis and Treatment, Beijing Anzhen Hospital, Capital Medical University, Beijing, China

Yang Gao Department of Radiology, Fuwai Hospital, Chinese Academy of Medical Sciences and Peking Union Medical College, Beijing, China

Zhihui Hou Department of Radiology, Fuwai Hospital, Chinese Academy of Medical Sciences and Peking Union Medical College, Beijing, China

Zheng-yu Jin Department of Radiology, Peking Union Medical College Hospital, Chinese Academy of Medical Sciences and Peking Union Medical College, Beijing, China

Lu Lin Department of Radiology, Peking Union Medical College Hospital, Chinese Academy of Medical Sciences and Peking Union Medical College, Beijing, China

Jia Liu Radiology Department, Peking University First Hospital, Beijing, China

Peijun Liu Department of Radiology, Peking Union Medical College Hospital, Chinese Academy of Medical Sciences and Peking Union Medical College, Beijing, China

Xiao Li Department of Radiology, Peking Union Medical College Hospital, Chinese Academy of Medical Sciences and Peking Union Medical College, Beijing, China

Bin Lu Department of Radiology, Fuwai Hospital, Chinese Academy of Medical Sciences and Peking Union Medical College, Beijing, China

Song Luo Department of Medical Imaging, Jinling Hospital, Medical School of Nanjing University, Nanjing, Jiangsu, China

Xinshuang Ren Department of Radiology, Fuwai Hospital, Chinese Academy of Medical Sciences and Peking Union Medical College, Beijing, China

Jian Wang Department of Radiology, Peking Union Medical College Hospital, Chinese Academy of Medical Sciences and Peking Union Medical College, Beijing, China

Rui Wang Radiology Department, Peking University First Hospital, Beijing, China

Yining Wang Department of Radiology, Peking Union Medical College Hospital, Chinese Academy of Medical Sciences and Peking Union Medical College, Beijing, China

Cheng Xu Department of Radiology, Peking Union Medical College Hospital, Chinese Academy of Medical Sciences and Peking Union Medical College, Beijing, China

Fan Yang Radiology Department, Tianjin Medical University General Hospital, Tianjin, China

Wei-hua Yin Department of Radiology, Fuwai Hospital, Chinese Academy of Medical Sciences and Peking Union Medical College, Beijing, China

Yan Yi Department of Radiology, Peking Union Medical College Hospital, Chinese Academy of Medical Sciences and Peking Union Medical College, Beijing, China

Yitong Yu Department of Radiology, Fuwai Hospital, Chinese Academy of Medical Sciences and Peking Union Medical College, Beijing, China

Zhang Zhang Radiology Department, Tianjin Medical University General Hospital, Tianjin, China

Kai Zhao Radiology Department, Peking University First Hospital, Beijing, China

Na Zhao Department of Radiology, Fuwai Hospital, Chinese Academy of Medical Sciences and Peking Union Medical College, Beijing, China

Fan Zhou Department of Medical Imaging, Jinling Hospital, Medical School of Nanjing University, Nanjing, Jiangsu, China

Kang Zhou Department of Radiology, Peking Union Medical College Hospital, Chinese Academy of Medical Sciences and Peking Union Medical College, Beijing, China

Abbreviations

AAA	Abdominal aortic aneurysm
AAOCA	Anomalous aortic origin of a coronary artery
AAOLCA	The left coronary arising from the right sinus of Valsalva
AAORCA	The right coronary arising from the left sinus of Valsalva
AAS	Acute Aortic Syndrome
ACS	Acute coronary syndrome
AD	Aortic dissection
AML	Anterior mitral leaflet
APVC	Anomalous pulmonary venous connections
ARVC	Arrhythmogenic right ventricular cardiomyopathy
ASA	Alcohol septal ablation
ASD	Atrial septal defect
ATP	Adenosine triphosphate
BP	Blood pressure
CA	Coronary angiography
CA	Carbohydrate antigen
CABG	Coronary artery bypass grafting
CAC	Coronary artery calcium
CACO	Coronary artery orinin anomalies
CACS	Coronary artery calcium score
CAD	Coronary artery disease
CAF	Coronary artery fistula
CCTA	Coronary computed tomography angiography
CHD	Congenital heart disease
CM	Cardiac myxoma
CMR	Cardiac magnetic resonance
CMRI	Cardiac magnetic resonance imaging
CPR	Curved multi-planar reformats
CRP	C-reactive protein
CT	Computed Tomographic
CTA	Computed tomography angiography
CT-FFR	Fractional flow reserve derived from CCTA
CTP	Myocardial CT perfusion
CTPA	Computed tomography pulmonary angiography
CXR	Chest-X-ray
D1	First diagonal branch
DCM	Hypertrophic cardiomyopathy

DE	Dual energy
DECT	Dual-energy CT
DES	Drug eluting stent
DORV	Double outlet right ventricle
DSA	Digital subtraction angiography
ECG	Electrocardiograph
ECV	Extracellular volume
EDV	End-diastolic volume
EF	Ejection fraction
ESC	European Society of Cardiology
ESR	Erythrocyte sedimentation rate
EULAR	European League Against Rheumatism)
EVAR	Endovascular Aortic Repair
FDG	Fluorodeoxyglucose
FDP	Fibrin Degradation product
FFR	Fractional flow reserve
FFRCT	Fractional flow reserve derived from CT
FL	Flase lumen
FOV	Field of view
HCM	Hypertrophic cardiomyopathy
HR	Heart rate
ICA	Invasive coronary angiography
IMA	Internal mammary artery
IMH	Intramural hematoma
ISR	In-stent restenosis
IVUS	Intravascular ultrasound
keV	Kiloelectron voltage
LA	Left atrial
LAD	Left anterior descending artery
LCX	Left circumflex artery
LGE	Late gadolinium enhancement
LL	Lesion length
LM	Left main artery
LV	Left ventricle
LV	Left ventricular
LVEF	Left ventricular ejection fraction
LVOTO	Left ventricular outflow tract obstruction
MBF	Myocardial blood flow
MBV	Myocardial blood volume
MCA	Mural coronary artery
MDCT	Multidetector computed tomography
MDT	Multidisciplinary team
MI	Myocardial infarction
MIBG	Metaiodobenzylguanidine
MIP	Maximum intensity projection
MPR	Multi-planar reformats
MR	Magnetic resonance
MRA	Magnetic resonance angiography

MRI	Magnetic resonance imaging
MSCT	Multislice spiral CT
NCPV	Non-calcified plaque volumes
NSTEMI	Non-ST-segment elevation myocardial infarction
OCT	Optical coherence tomography
PCI	Percutaneous coronary intervention
PDA	Posterior descending artery
PDA	Patent ductus arteriosus
PET	Positron emission tomography
PL	Posterolateral
PM	Papillary muscle
PS	Pulmonary stenosis
RA	Right atrium
RCA	Right coronary artery
RCM	Restrictive cardiomyopathy
RI	Remodeling index
RV	Right ventricular
RVOT	Right ventricular outflow tract
SAM	Systolic anterior motion
SCD	Sudden cardiac death
SE	Spin echo
SPECT	Single photon emission computed tomography
STEMI	ST-segment elevation myocardial infarction
STJ	Sinotubular junction
SVG	Saphenous vein grafts
TAA	Thoracic aortic aneurysm
TAD	Thoracic aortic dissection
TAG	Transluminal attenuation gradient
TAK	Takayasu's arteritis
TEE	Transesophageal echocardiography
TEVAR	Thoracic Endovascular Aortic Repair
TL	True lunmen
TOF	Tetralogy of fallot
TPS	Tissue polypeptide specific antigen
TTE	Transthoracic echocardiogram
TVI	Tricuspid inflow velocity
UCG	Echocardiography
VMI	Virtual monoenergetic images
VMI	Virtual monoenergetic imaging
VNC	Virtual noncontrast
VNC	Virtual non-enhancement
VNC	Virtual non-contrast
VR	Volume rendering
VSD	Ventricular septal defect
WBC	White blood cell

Reversible Myocardial Ischemia

Yan Yi, Yining Wang, and Zheng-yu Jin

Abstract

Reversible myocardial ischemia is a common disease that occurs in patients with atherosclerosis of coronary artery, myocardial microcirculation disturbance, and other infrequent etiologies. It is mainly due to the blood perfusion insufficiency of the myocardium. Ischemia is the single most important predictor of future hard cardiac events and ischemia correction remains the cornerstone of current revascularization strategies (Kennedy MW, Fabris E, Suryapranata H, Kedhi E, Cardiovasc Diabetol 16:51, 2017). Early accurate diagnosis of reversible myocardial ischemia is of great importance for reducing the incidence of myocardial infarction and improving the prognosis of patients. The electrocardiogram (ECG), functional testing, cardiac stress test (including exercise stress test and pharmacological stress test), and myocardial perfusion imaging were all the methods of choice for detecting myocardial ischemia. Among all these methods, the myocardial perfusion imaging approaches, which traditionally consist of radionuclide myocardial perfusion and magnetic resonance (MR) myocardial perfusion, have been considered as effective and accurate. Recently, with the rapid development of CT imaging techniques, CT myocardial perfusion imaging has been demonstrated as a promising noninvasive diagnostic strategy for myocardial ischemia. Up to now, the invasive fractional flow reserve (FFR) has been regarded as the "gold standard" for diagnosing hemodynamically significant coronary artery disease (CAD). In this chapter, based on a case of reversible myocardial ischemia, we will discuss the cardiac CT imaging manifestations of myocardial ischemia, and further possibly promising role of new cardiac CT technology, particularly the CT myocardial perfusion, in reversible myocardial ischemia.

1.1 Case of Reversible Myocardial Ischemia

1.1.1 History

- A 66-year-old male patient felt intermittent shortness of breath for more than 2 months, which can be relieved by deep breathing.
- He was appointed to coronary CT angiography and myocardial CT perfusion imaging for suspected CAD.

1.1.1.1 Physical Examination
- Blood pressure: 160/95 mmHg; Breathing rate: 17/min.
- Heart rate: 64 bpm without arrhythmia.
- No pathological murmurs were detected in the auscultation area.

Y. Yi · Y. Wang · Z.-y. Jin (✉)
Department of Radiology, Peking Union Medical College Hospital, Chinese Academy of Medical Sciences and Peking Union Medical College, Beijing, China
e-mail: jinzy@pumch.cn

© Springer Nature Singapore Pte Ltd. 2020
Z.-y. Jin et al. (eds.), *Cardiac CT*, https://doi.org/10.1007/978-981-15-5305-9_1

1.1.1.2 Electrocardiograph

Standard 12 lead ECG revealed sinus rhythm, PR 0.914 s, ST-T segment elevated 0.1mv on leads V2.

1.1.1.3 Laboratory

Serum myocardial enzyme spectrum showed negative results.

1.1.2 Imaging Examination

1.1.2.1 CT Images

A coronary CT angiography (CTA) combined with adenosine triphosphate (ATP)-stress myocardial CT perfusion was requested to investigate the coronary artery status and myocardial blood flow (Figs. 1.1, 1.2, and 1.3).

1.1.2.2 Conventional Coronary Angiography and FFR (Fig. 1.4)

1.1.3 Imaging Findings and Diagnosis

The coronary CTA images results showed there were mixed plaques in the proximal segments of LAD and D1, resulting in moderate to severe lumen stenosis. However, the severe calcified plaques on the CTA images make it difficult to assess the lesion accurately. In addition, the evaluation of CTA was limited to morphological information. After the imaging of myocardial CT perfusion, results of bull-eye polar-maps and two-short chamber views demonstrated the reduction of myocardial blood flow in the anterior wall of left ventricular myocardium without delayed enhancement, which means there was reversible myocardial ischemia corresponding to

the coronary blood supply region of lesion vessels. The invasive coronary angiography (ICA) images and FFR result confirmed the hemodynamically significant CAD.

1.1.4 Management

- Conventional medical therapy for Secondary Prevention of CAD
- Out-patient follow-up observations for CAD with reversible myocardial ischemia

1.2 Discussion

Reversible myocardial ischemia is one of the most common diseases, which most often occurs in patients with CAD. This mainly results from the hemodynamically significant coronary stenosis. The common clinical symptoms include slight chest tightness, stable effort angina (chest tightness, palpitations, shortness of breath, exercising and anxious prone, self-relief during rest), and rest pain (during rest state or sleeping).

Prompt accurate diagnosis of reversible myocardial ischemia has important significance in helping not only guiding downstream decision-making for medical therapy versus revascularization and PCI versus CABG, but also evaluating clinical prognosis. Clinically, ECG is a mostly practical and convenient method, yet it is unable to provide comprehensive information and sometimes may not be accurate. Functional and cardiac stress tests are other approaches for myocardial ischemia detection; however, some patients are not capable of cooperating satisfactorily.

In recent decades, myocardial perfusion imaging is being recognized as a most direct and accu-

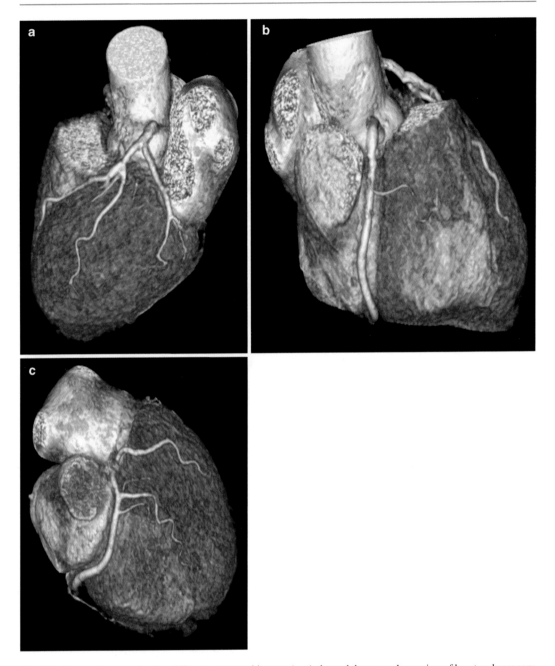

Fig. 1.1 Volumetric reproduction (VR) reconstructed images (**a–c**) showed the general overview of heart and coronary arteries. ((**a**) Left anterior descending (LAD) branch and left circumflex artery (LCx) (**b–c**) right coronary artery (RCA))

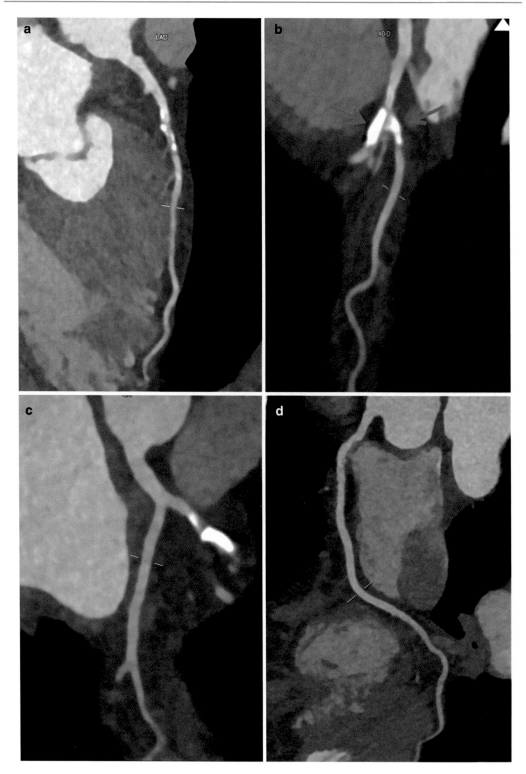

Fig. 1.2 Curved multi-planar reformats (MPR) reconstructed images of the coronary arteries (**a, b**, left anterior descending [LAD] branch and First diagonal branch (D1); (**c**) left circumflex artery [LCx]; (**d**) right coronary artery [RCA]). There were mixed plaques in the proximal segment of LAD and D1. With severe calcification, the stenosis of the lumen was difficult to evaluate accurately

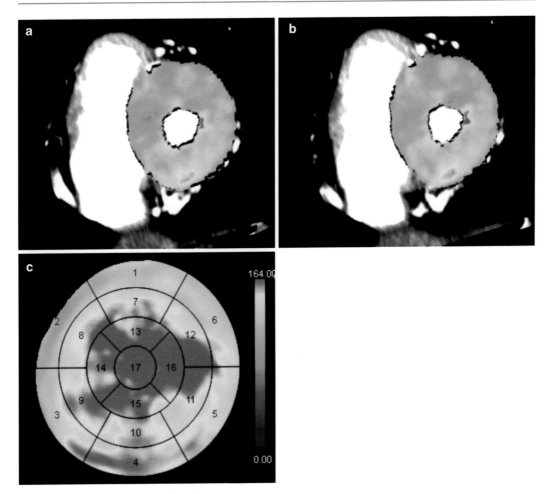

Fig. 1.3 Cardiac CT perfusion imaging of myocardium of short-axis two-chamber view (**a, b**) of left ventricular and myocardial blood flow (MBF) pseudo-color images of Bull-eye polar-map (**c**), both showed the blood perfusion reduction in the anterior wall of left ventricular myocardium

rate method for indicating myocardial ischemia. Based on a relatively long development period, the radionuclide myocardial perfusion and MR myocardial perfusion are most commonly utilized in our clinical practice. Both of them can evaluate the myocardial blood perfusion situation on per-segment, per-vessel, and per-patient basement. Nevertheless, there are still some limitations for these two approaches: the implementation of radionuclide myocardial perfusion is inevitably related to radiation dose, and the sensitivity was relatively inferior to MR perfusion imaging; while MR imaging has some contraindications for patients, like claustrophobia or with recent stent implantation. In the last decade, with the

rapid development of CT imaging techniques, myocardial CT perfusion has come into people's vision, and it has been demonstrated as a promising noninvasive diagnostic strategy for myocardial ischemia.

Up to now, the invasive FFR has been regarded as the "gold standard" for diagnosing hemodynamically significant CAD. The FFR also has been regarded as "gold standard" for guiding downstream decision-making to decide if the revascularization is needed or not.

Generally, if the patients received timely and accurate diagnosis and treatment, the ischemia can be reversed and a favorable prognosis could be expected. Otherwise, reversible myocardial

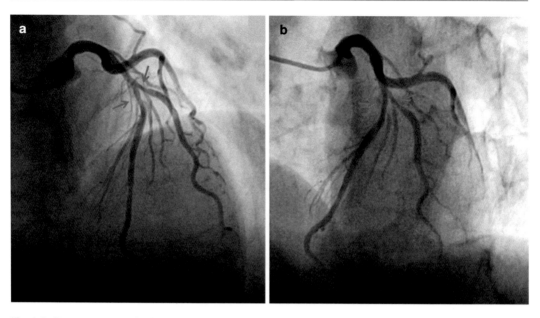

Fig. 1.4 Percutaneous transluminal coronary intervention (PCI) results. Invasive coronary angiography image of LAD and D1, (**a**, **b**, red arrow) with the corresponding FFR results lower than 0.8

ischemia may develop into myocardial infarction, which is irreversible and the prognosis may be poor.

1.3 Current Technical Status and Applications of CT

Radionuclide myocardial perfusion and MR perfusion imaging were most commonly utilized for diagnosing myocardial ischemia in our traditional daily practice. However, during the development of the last few decades, new technologies like single-energy first-pass CT acquisition, dual-energy (DE) CCTA, and myocardial perfusion imaging have become more and more popular as noninvasive medical imaging methods for evaluating hemodynamically significant CAD [1].

The single-energy first-pass CT allows static assessment of myocardial blood pool [2]. Multiple studies have shown that the rest and stress first-pass CT may be able to identify the myocardial ischemia with the reference standard of ICA, single photon emission computed tomography (SPECT), or MR. [3–7] Yet the challenge is a relatively subtle attenuation difference in the areas of perfusion defects.

The dual-energy first-pass CT also has been demonstrated capable of static assessment of myocardial blood pool as single-energy first-pass CT. However, on the basis of energy spectrum analysis, it was more advantaged for quantitatively detecting the myocardial ischemia. DE static first-pass CT makes mapping of iodine distribution possible, which in turn serves as a surrogate for myocardial perfusion [2]. Previous studies have documented enhanced tissue differentiation, along with high image quality and improved accuracy for detection of CAD using DECT imaging [8]. As tissue attenuation profiles obtained at two different energy levels, the disparity in energy-related absorption properties between the two X-ray spectra utilized in DECT allows for one to distinguish materials of sufficiently diverse attenuation profiles. Research has [9] demonstrated that monochromatic DECT imaging at 40 keV exhibited a higher diagnostic performance as compared with material density imaging using iodine-muscle basis pairs for the detection of myocardial ischemia as defined by perfusion defects detected with SPECT.

Comparing to SPECT and MR, with higher temporal and spatial resolution and development of radiation dose reduction, stress dynamic myocardial CT perfusion has emerged as a potential method for evaluation of hemodynamic myocardial ischemia in the clinical application [10]. It can be organized as a preoperative examination to investigate MBF, myocardial blood volume (MBV) and so on. Additional myocardial CT perfusion imaging may be helpful to identify patients with myocardial ischemia in whom coronary revascularization therapy would be beneficial [11]. A systematic review and meta-analysis have shown that stress dynamic myocardial CT perfusion has a high diagnostic accuracy in detecting myocardial ischemia and it may increase significantly at segment level in the combined use of coronary CTA [10]. Lately, a research even showed that single-phase CCTA can be extracted from stress dynamic myocardial CT perfusion for coronary artery stenosis assessment. The image quality and diagnostic value of single-phase CCTA were equivalent to routine CCTA on third-generation dual-source CT, which potentially allows the possibility of "one-stop" cardiac examination for high-risk CAD patients who need myocardial ischemia assessment [12].

As we can expect, myocardial CT perfusion is ready for clinical use for detecting myocardial ischemia caused by obstructive disease. Nevertheless, the clinical utility of CT perfusion to identify ischemia in patients with nonobstructive/microvascular disease still has to be established [11].

Lately, the FFR derived from CT (FFRCT) has shown its potential value for CAD patients with hemodynamically significant stenosis. It offers a noninvasive method for evaluating the borderline stenosis based on computational fluid dynamics calculation [13] or machine learning technology [14]. Both methods outperform the accuracy of coronary CTA and ICA in the detection of flow-limiting stenosis.

Integrating studies of myocardial CT perfusion and FFRCT in the work-up of CAD showed that both of them identify functionally significant CAD with comparable accuracy. Diagnostic performance can be improved by combining these two techniques. A stepwise approach, reserving myocardial CT perfusion for intermediate FFRCT results, also improves diagnostic performance while omitting nearly one-half of the population from myocardial CT perfusion examinations [15].

As we can see, appropriate cardiac CT examination contributes a lot for guiding downstream decision-making of treatment and evaluating clinical prognosis.

1.4 Key Points

- Reversible myocardial ischemia is one of the most clinical conditions in CAD patients.
- Multiple imaging approaches are capable of identifying myocardial ischemia, which is related to the hemodynamically significant coronary stenosis.
- Myocardial perfusion and fractional flow reserve derived from CT are the two most appropriate cardiac CT imaging methods for detecting hemodynamically CAD.

References

1. Yi Y, Jin ZY, Wang YN. Advances in myocardial CT perfusion imaging technology. Am J Transl Res. 2016;8(11):4523–31.
2. Bucher AM, De Cecco CN, Schoepf UJ, Wang R, Meinel FG, Binukrishnan SR, et al. Cardiac CT for myocardial ischaemia detection and characterization--comparative analysis. Br J Radiol. 2014;87(1043):20140159. https://doi.org/10.1259/bjr.20140159.
3. Nagao M, Matsuoka H, Kawakami H, Higashino H, Mochizuki T, Ohshita A, et al. Detection of myocardial ischemia using 64-slice MDCT. Circ J. 2009;73(5):905–11. https://doi.org/10.1253/circj.cj-08-0940.
4. Gupta M, Kadakia J, Jug B, Mao SS, Budoff MJ. Detection and quantification of myocardial perfusion defects by resting single-phase 64-slice cardiac computed tomography angiography compared with SPECT myocardial perfusion imaging. Coron Artery Dis. 2013;24(4):290–7. https://doi.org/10.1097/MCA.0b013e32835f2fe5.
5. Nikolaou K, Sanz J, Poon M, Wintersperger BJ, Ohnesorge B, Rius T, et al. Assessment of myocardial perfusion and viability from routine contrast-enhanced 16-detector-row computed tomography of the heart: preliminary results. Eur Radiol. 2005;15(5):864–71. https://doi.org/10.1007/s00330-005-2672-6.
6. Iwasaki K, Matsumoto T. Myocardial perfusion defect in patients with coronary artery disease dem-

onstrated by 64-multidetector computed tomography at rest. Clin Cardiol. 2011;34(7):454–60. https://doi.org/10.1002/clc.20908.

7. Kachenoura N, Lodato JA, Gaspar T, Bardo DM, Newby B, Gips S, et al. Value of multidetector computed tomography evaluation of myocardial perfusion in the assessment of ischemic heart disease: comparison with nuclear perfusion imaging. Eur Radiol. 2009;19(8):1897–905. https://doi.org/10.1007/s00330-009-1365-y.

8. Scheske JA, O'Brien JM, Earls JP, Min JK, LaBounty TM, Cury RC, et al. Coronary artery imaging with single-source rapid kilovolt peak-switching dual-energy CT. Radiology. 2013;268(3):702–9. https://doi.org/10.1148/radiol.13121901.

9. Danad I, Cho I, Elmore K, Schulman-Marcus J, Óhartaigh B, Stuijfzand WJ, et al. Comparative diagnostic accuracy of dual-energy CT myocardial perfusion imaging by monochromatic energy versus material decomposition methods. Clin Imaging. 2018;50:1–4. https://doi.org/10.1016/j.clinimag.2017.11.002.

10. Lu M, Wang S, Sirajuddin A, Arai AE, Zhao S. Dynamic stress computed tomography myocardial perfusion for detecting myocardial ischemia: a systematic review and meta-analysis. Int J Cardiol. 2018;258:325–31. https://doi.org/10.1016/j.ijcard.2018.01.095.

11. Takx RAP, Celeng C, Schoepf UJ. CT myocardial perfusion imaging: ready for prime time? Eur Radiol. 2018;28(3):1253–6. https://doi.org/10.1007/s00330-017-5057-8.

12. Yi Y, Wu W, Lin L, Zhang HZ, Qian H, Shen ZJ, et al. Single-phase coronary artery CT angiography extracted from stress dynamic myocardial CT perfusion on third-generation dual-source CT: validation by coronary angiography. Int J Cardiol. 2018;269:343–9. https://doi.org/10.1016/j.ijcard.2018.06.112.

13. Min JK, Taylor CA, Achenbach S, Koo BK, Leipsic J, Norgaard BL, et al. Noninvasive fractional flow reserve derived from coronary CT angiography: clinical data and scientific principles. JACC Cardiovasc Imaging. 2015;8(10):1209–22. https://doi.org/10.1016/j.jcmg.2015.08.006.

14. Tesche C, De Cecco CN, Baumann S, Renker M, McLaurin TW, Duguay TM, et al. Coronary CT angiography-derived fractional flow reserve: machine learning algorithm versus computational fluid dynamics modeling. Radiology. 2018;288(1):64–72. https://doi.org/10.1148/radiol.2018171291.

15. Coenen A, Rossi A, Lubbers MM, Kurata A, Kono AK, Chelu RG, et al. Integrating CT myocardial perfusion and CT-FFR in the work-up of coronary artery disease. JACC Cardiovasc Imaging. 2017;10(7):760–70. https://doi.org/10.1016/j.jcmg.2016.09.028.

Myocardial Infarction

2

Peijun Liu, Yining Wang, and Zheng-yu Jin

Abstract

Myocardial infarction (MI) is myocardial necrosis caused by myocardial ischemia. Pathologically, it is defined as myocardial cell death due to prolonged myocardial ischemia. Noninvasive imaging plays an important role in diagnosing known or suspected MI. Echocardiography and cardiac magnetic resonance imaging (CMRI) are used to assess cardiac structure and function, especially myocardial thickness and motion. Late enhancement in CMRI is associated with myocardial fibrosis and indicates the presence and extent of MI. Radionuclide imaging is the only commonly available method for evaluating myocardial viability and myocardial metabolism directly. Recently, the latest advances in CT scanner technique have opened a new era for cardiac imaging with MI patients. In this chapter, we will describe the characteristics of MI in cardiac CT imaging, and further discuss the application of new cardiac CT technology in patients with MI.

2.1 Case of MI

2.1.1 History

A 50-year-old male patient came to our hospital for routine physical examination without syndrome. He had hypertension for 10 years and a family history of coronary artery disease (CAD).

2.1.1.1 Physical Examination
- Blood pressure: 131/94 mmHg
- Breathing rate: 18/min
- Heart rate: 65 bpm without arrhythmia

2.1.1.2 Laboratory
The level of troponin is 1.205 µg/L.

2.1.2 Imaging Examination

2.1.2.1 CT Images
Coronary CT angiography and delay enhancement were performed to evaluate coronary artery and myocardium (Figs. 2.1 and 2.2).

P. Liu · Y. Wang · Z.-y. Jin (✉)
Department of Radiology, Peking Union Medical College Hospital, Chinese Academy of Medical Sciences and Peking Union Medical College, Beijing, China
e-mail: jinzy@pumch.cn

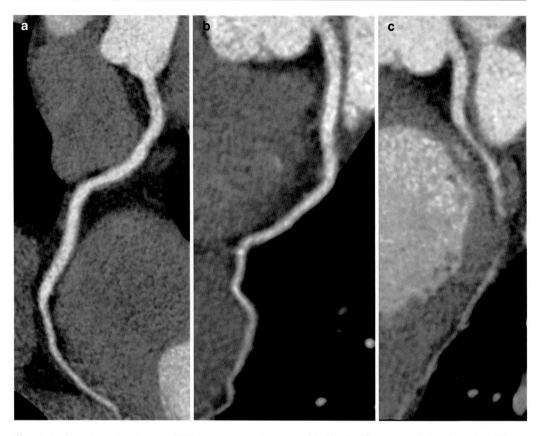

Fig. 2.1 Curved multi-planar (CPR) reconstructed images of the coronary CTA showed severe stenosis to occlusion at the proximal and middle left circumflex artery (**c**). No significant stenosis has been found in the left anterior descending artery (**a**) and right coronary artery (**b**)

2.1.2.2 Conventional Coronary Angiography (Fig. 2.3)

2.1.2.3 MRI Images (Fig. 2.4)

2.1.3 Imaging Findings and Diagnosis

At standard coronary CT angiography, 40-keV virtual monochromatic image and iodine density map showed focal hypo-enhancement in the inferolateral myocardial wall, which was corresponding to the left circumflex artery territory. Suspected myocardial ischemia existed in this area. Iodine density map showed an iodine content of 0.6 mg/mL in the suspected myocardial ischemia segment and an iodine content of 2.0 mg/mL in the remote normal myocardial segment. At late iodine enhancement imaging, the corresponding area (inferolateral myocardial wall) revealed focal transmural delay enhancement at 40-keV virtual monochromatic image and iodine density map, which showed clearly infarcted myocardium. Iodine density map in this stage found an iodine content of 2.2 mg/mL in the delay enhanced segment and an iodine content of 1.2 mg/mL in the remote unaffected myocardial segment. ECV calculated from the iodine density map for the infarcted and remote normal segments were 53% and 29%, respectively, which indicated severe myocardial fibrosis in the infarcted segment.

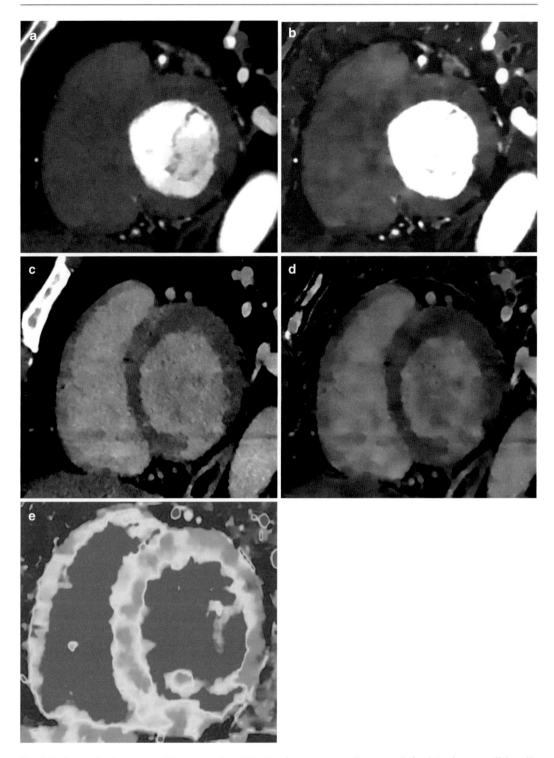

Fig. 2.2 At standard coronary CT angiography, 40-keV virtual monochromatic image (**a**) and iodine density map (**b**) showed focal hypo-enhancement in the inferolateral myocardial wall, which was corresponding to the left circumflex artery territory. At late iodine enhancement imaging, corresponding area (inferolateral myocardial wall) revealed focal delay enhancement at 40-keV virtual monochromatic image (**c**) and iodine density map (**d**). The extracellular volume (ECV) for the infarcted and remote normal segments were 53% and 29%, respectively (**e**)

2.1.4 Management

- Percutaneous coronary intervention operation therapy
- Conventional medical therapy for CAD

2.2 Discussion

MI is an event of heart attack due to an imbalance between oxygen supply and myocardial demand resulting in myocardial injury. According to elec-

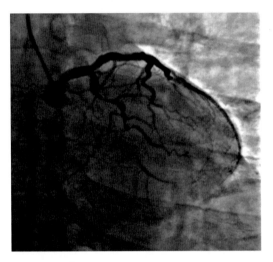

Fig. 2.3 Percutaneous coronary intervention showed severe stenosis to occlusion at the proximal and middle left circumflex artery

trocardiogram trace, MI is differentiated between non-ST-segment elevation myocardial infarction (NSTEMI) and ST-segment elevation myocardial infarction (STEMI). STEMI is the result of transmural myocardial ischemia that involves the full thickness of the myocardium, while NSTEMI does not spread across all the myocardial wall [1]. STEMI, NSTEMI, and unstable angina pectoris are formed in the concept of acute coronary syndrome [2]. The clinical symptoms of MI include chest and upper extremity diffuse discomfort, fatigue and shortness of breath during exertion or at rest. However, about 64% of people with MI have no obvious symptom, which is called silent MI [3].

Noninvasive imaging acts as an important role in diagnosing and characterizing MI. Regional and global wall motion abnormalities induced by myocardial ischemia can be observed by echocardiography and CMRI. Tissue Doppler and strain imaging from echocardiography are used for quantification of regional and global function. Radionuclide imaging allows assessing myocardial viability and myocardial metabolism by radionuclide tracers. CMRI has the ability to assess myocardial perfusion and myocardial fibrosis of MI. In addition, CMRI also allows detection of the presence and extent of myocardial edema or inflammation to distinct acute or chronic MI.

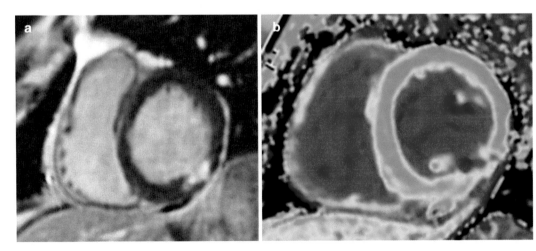

Fig. 2.4 Cardiac magnetic resonance imaging showed transmural lateral late gadolinium enhancement in the inferolateral myocardial wall (**a**). ECV in the infarcted and remote unaffected segments were 50% and 23%, respectively (**b**)

2.3 Current Technical Status and Applications of CT

Compared with invasive coronary angiography, conventional CT angiography has an advantage in assessing coronary stenosis with 95–99% sensitivity and 97–99% specificity [4]. However, myocardial analysis is limited by motion and beam-hardening artifacts [5]. With the advance of CT technique, dual-energy CT open new era for cardiac imaging in which attenuation data from different energies are used to characterize material properties. CT perfusion imaging, late iodine enhancement CT imaging, and CT strain imaging are now used for analyzing myocardial function.

Dual-energy CT technique not only corrects beam-hardening artifacts to improve image quality, but also generates iodine map to increase accuracy in evaluating MI. Iodine map reflects the distribution of iodine in myocardium, which is correlated with myocardial perfusion and blood flow [6]. CT perfusion imaging is used for evaluating fixed and reversible perfusion defects with myocardial injury. Qualitative and quantitative analysis can be obtained from myocardial perfusion imaging. In addition, the combination of coronary analysis and myocardial perfusion imaging provides a significant incremental value over coronary CT angiography alone for the detection of hemodynamically significant stenosis in CAD patients [7].

CMRI is used as the reference standard for evaluation of myocardial fibrosis or scarring. Meanwhile, myocardial extracellular volume fraction acquired from CMRI is now considered a reliable parameter for the assessment of diffuse myocardial fibrosis [8]. However, late iodine enhancement CT imaging is an alternative approach to late gadolinium enhancement MRI because the pharmacokinetics of iodinated contrast materials are similar to those of gadolinium-containing contrast materials [9]. Virtual monoenergetic from dual-energy CT can improve the image quality of late iodine enhancement [10]. In addition, myocardial ECV with dual-energy CT has good agreement and excellent correlation with MR ECV imaging [11, 12].

Myocardial strain imaging has emerged as a quantitative approach to assess regional cardiac function using cardiac CT [13]. Conventional myocardial strain imaging allows identification of MI by the degree of two-dimensional (2D) strain reduction, which mainly measured strain of three orthogonal directions of myocardial motion: longitudinal strain, circumferential strain, and radial strain. Recently, three-dimensional maximum principal strain acquired from cardiac CT can also be used for detecting regional cardiac dysfunction with MI [14].

Technological advancements in CT imaging have extended more potential for assessment of MI than conventional CT image, which is helpful for disease identification and clinical management.

2.4 Key Points

- The combination of coronary CTA with CT perfusion/late iodine enhancement imaging provides comprehensive information for patients with MI.
- New CT techniques offer more advantages than conventional CT techniques, particularly for myocardial viability analysis.

References

1. Vogel B, Claessen BE, Arnold SV, Chan D, Cohen DJ, Giannitsis E, et al. ST-segment elevation myocardial infarction. Nat Rev Dis Primers. 2019;5(1):39. https://doi.org/10.1038/s41572-019-0090-3.
2. Amsterdam EA, Wenger NK, Brindis RG, Casey DE, Ganiats TG, Holmes DR, et al. 2014 AHA/ACC guideline for the management of patients with non-ST-elevation acute coronary syndromes: a report of the American College of Cardiology/American Heart Association Task Force on Practice Guidelines. Circulation. 2014;130(25):e344–426. https://doi.org/10.1161/cir.0000000000000134.
3. Valensi P, Lorgis L, Cottin Y. Prevalence, incidence, predictive factors and prognosis of silent myocardial infarction: a review of the literature. Arch Cardiovasc Dis. 2011;104(3):178–88. https://doi.org/10.1016/j.acvd.2010.11.013.
4. Hamon M, Biondi-Zoccai GG, Malagutti P, Agostoni P, Morello R, Valgimigli M, et al. Diagnostic performance of multislice spiral computed tomography

of coronary arteries as compared with conventional invasive coronary angiography: a meta-analysis. J Am Coll Cardiol. 2006;48(9):1896–910. https://doi.org/10.1016/j.jacc.2006.08.028.

5. Kalisz K, Halliburton S, Abbara S, Leipsic JA, Albrecht MH, Schoepf UJ, et al. Update on cardiovascular applications of multienergy CT. Radiographics. 2017;37(7):1955–74. https://doi.org/10.1148/rg.2017170100.

6. Danad I, Fayad ZA, Willemink MJ, Min JK. New applications of cardiac computed tomography: dual-energy, spectral, and molecular CT imaging. J Am Coll Cardiol Img. 2015;8(6):710–23. https://doi.org/10.1016/j.jcmg.2015.03.005.

7. Carrascosa PM, Deviggiano A, Capunay C, Campisi R, López de Munain M, Vallejos J, et al. Incremental value of myocardial perfusion over coronary angiography by spectral computed tomography in patients with intermediate to high likelihood of coronary artery disease. Eur J Radiol. 2015;84(4):637–42. https://doi.org/10.1016/j.ejrad.2014.12.013.

8. Messroghli DR, Moon JC, Ferreira VM, Grosse-Wortmann L, He T, Kellman P, et al. Clinical recommendations for cardiovascular magnetic resonance mapping of T1, T2, T2∗ and extracellular volume: a consensus statement by the Society for Cardiovascular Magnetic Resonance (SCMR) endorsed by the European Association for Cardiovascular Imaging (EACVI). J Cardiovasc Magn Reson. 2017;19(1):75. https://doi.org/10.1186/s12968-017-0389-8.

9. Schuleri KH, George RT, Lardo AC. Applications of cardiac multidetector CT beyond coronary angiography. Nat Rev Cardiol. 2009;6(11):699–710. https://doi.org/10.1038/nrcardio.2009.172.

10. Wichmann JL, Arbaciauskaite R, Kerl JM, Frellesen C, Bodelle B, Lehnert T, et al. Evaluation of monoenergetic late iodine enhancement dual-energy computed tomography for imaging of chronic myocardial infarction. Eur Radiol. 2014;24(6):1211–8. https://doi.org/10.1007/s00330-014-3126-9.

11. Lee HJ, Im DJ, Youn JC, Chang S, Suh YJ, Hong YJ, et al. Myocardial extracellular volume fraction with dual-energy equilibrium contrast-enhanced cardiac CT in nonischemic cardiomyopathy: a prospective comparison with cardiac MR imaging. Radiology. 2016;280(1):49–57. https://doi.org/10.1148/radiol.2016151289.

12. Oda S, Emoto T, Nakaura T, Kidoh M, Utsunomiya D, Funama Y, et al. Myocardial late iodine enhancement and extracellular volume quantification with dual-layer spectral detector dual-energy cardiac CT. Radiology: Cardiothoracic Imaging. 2019;1(1):e180003. https://doi.org/10.1148/ryct.2019180003.

13. Tee M, Noble JA, Bluemke DA. Imaging techniques for cardiac strain and deformation: comparison of echocardiography, cardiac magnetic resonance and cardiac computed tomography. Expert Rev Cardiovasc Ther. 2013;11(2):221–31. https://doi.org/10.1586/erc.12.182.

14. Tanabe Y, Kido T, Kurata A, Sawada S, Suekuni H, Kido T, et al. Three-dimensional maximum principal strain using cardiac computed tomography for identification of myocardial infarction. Eur Radiol. 2017;27(4):1667–75. https://doi.org/10.1007/s00330-016-4550-9.

Coronary Artery In-Stent Restenosis

3

Cheng Xu and Yining Wang

Abstract

In-stent restenosis (ISR) is a common complication after coronary artery stent placement. Angiographic restenosis is defined as >50% diameter stenosis of the stented segment and clinically restenosis is defined as recurrence of clinical manifestations of ischemia. ISR is arising from neointimal hyperplasia and smooth muscle hypertrophy. The incidence of ISR at 6 months is around 25% after bare-metal stents implantation, and less than 10% after drug-eluting stents implantation. The gold standard to evaluate ISR is invasive coronary angiography, which is an invasive process. With the development of multidetector computed tomography (MDCT) image technology, CT has become a useful noninvasive modality for evaluating ISR. In this chapter, based on a case of ISR, we will discuss the CT imaging manifestations and accurate assessment of ISR, and further possibly promising role of CT technology in ISR.

3.1 Case of ISR

3.1.1 History

A 41-year-old female patient felt chest pain which relieved by rest for the past month. She had a history of PCI a year ago, four stents were implanted in the left main artery (LM), left anterior descending artery (LAD), right coronary artery (RCA), and right posterolateral (PL) artery, respectively. She was appointed to cardiac CT for suspected ISR or coronary artery disease (CAD) progression.

Physical Examination
- Blood pressure: 125/83 mmHg; breathing rate: 18/min
- Heart rate: 83 bpm, without arrhythmia

Electrocardiograph
Standard 12-lead electrocardiograph (ECG) revealed ST-T segment changes on leads aVR and aVL.

Laboratory
Serum myocardial enzyme spectrum showed negative results.

C. Xu · Y. Wang (✉)
Department of Radiology, Peking Union Medical College Hospital, Chinese Academy of Medical Sciences and Peking Union Medical College, Beijing, China
e-mail: wangyining@pumch.cn

3.1.2 Imaging Examination

CT Images
A coronary CT angiography (CTA) combined with adenosine triphosphate (ATP)-stress myocardial CT perfusion was performed (Figs. 3.1, 3.2, and 3.3).

Conventional Coronary Angiography (Fig. 3.4)

3.1.3 Imaging Findings and Diagnosis

The coronary CTA images results showed there was low density within the stented segment of LM and the in-stent lumen was obviously with stenosis, the in-stent lumen patency of mid-LAD was difficult to evaluate because of beam-hardening artifacts (B26f). The curved multi-planar reconstruction of LAD on sharp convolution kernel (B46f) showed low density within the stented segment of LAD more clearly. There were noncalcified plaques between the two stents of LAD, resulting in severe lumen stenosis. No significant stenosis or ISR had been found in RCA. Bull-eye polar-map, four-chamber view, and two-short chamber view showed the extensive reduction of myocardial blood flow in the anterior and anteroseptal myocardium compared to the basal area, which is corresponding to the coronary blood supply region of LAD. The angiography images confirmed ISR in LM and LAD.

3.1.4 Management

- Transluminal balloon dilatation of LM-LAD
- Stent implantation in the middle of LAD
- Conventional medical therapy for CAD

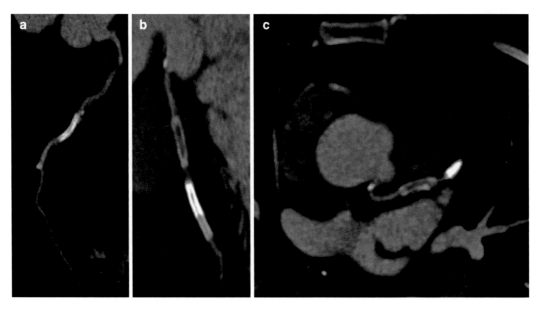

Fig. 3.1 Coronary CTA B26f. Curved multi-planar (CPR) reconstructed images (**a**, right coronary artery [RCA]; (**b**) left anterior descending artery [LAD]) and multiplane reconstruction (MPR) image (**c**) of the coronary CTA. Hypo-attenuation was found within the in-stent lumen of LM and the in-stent lumen was obviously with stenosis, the patency of the stented segment of mid-LAD was difficult to evaluate. Noncalcified plaque was found between two stents. There was no stenosis in the stent of RCA

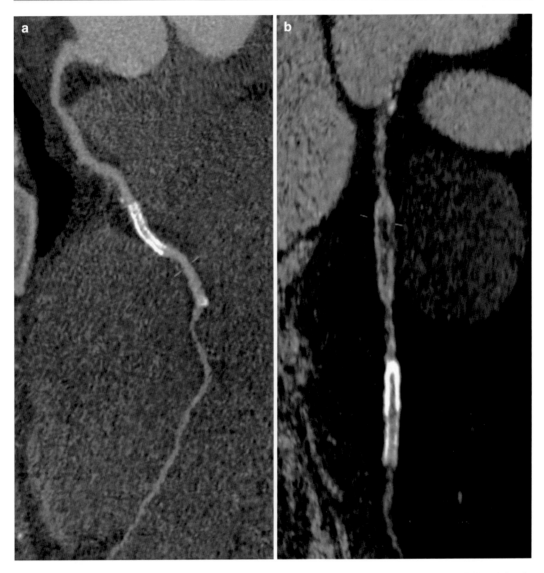

Fig. 3.2 Coronary CTA B46f. Curved multi-planar (CPR) reconstructed images (**a**, RCA; **b**, LAD). Filling defect in the stent of mid-LAD was clearly shown

3.2 Discussion

ISR can be divided into four types: I-focal, with length <10 mm and positioned at the proximal or distal margin; II-diffuse, with length >10 mm, not exceeding the edges of the stent; III-proliferative, length >10 mm, exceeding the edges of the stent; and IV-occlusive, total occlusion with TIMI (thrombolysis in myocardial infarction) 0 [1].

ICA is the gold standard for assessing ISR. Intravascular ultrasound (IVUS) allows for the assessment of all different cross-section of a vessel and provides detailed information about neointimal hyperplasia. Optical coherence tomography has higher resolution and provides more

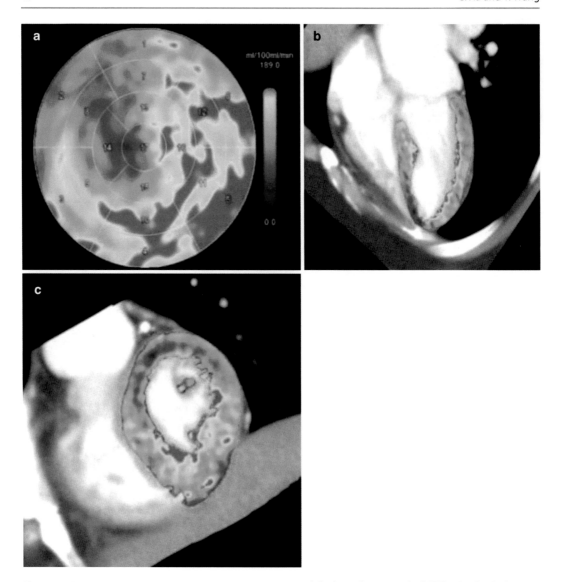

Fig. 3.3 CT perfusion myocardial blood flow (MBF) pseudo-color images: Bull-eye polar-map (**a**), four-chamber view (**b**), short-axis two-chamber view (**c**) of left ventricle showed an extensive MBF reduction in the anterior and anteroseptal myocardium compared to the basal segments

detailed information of the stented segment. CT is a noninvasive evaluation technique, ISR was identified by a darker area within the in-stent lumen, with a lumen decrease $\geq 50\%$. According to a meta-analysis, the specificity, sensitivity, positive predictive value, and negative predictive value of 64 multi-slice CT to diagnose ISR reached 90%, 91%, 68%, and 98%, respectively [2].

The presenting symptoms of ISR include stable angina, unstable angina, or myocardial infarction. The primary clinical manifestation is acute coronary syndrome (ACS, including unstable angina or myocardial infarction). For bare-metal stent, first-generation and second-generation drug-eluting stent, ACS account for 67.8%, 71.0%, and 66.7% of the clinical manifestation respectively [3].

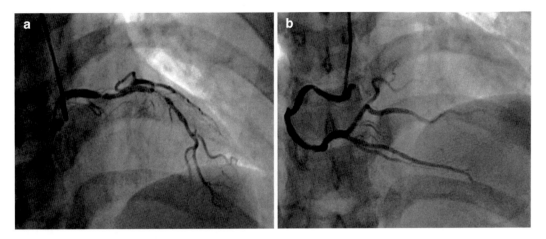

Fig. 3.4 Invasive coronary angiography image for LAD (**a**) and RCA (**b**). The result show in-stent restenosis in LM-LAD and there was no in-stent restenosis in RCA

3.3 Current Technical Status and Applications of CT

Coronary CTA has become increasingly used in the detection of in-stent restenosis during the follow-ups. A meta-analysis shows CTA could evaluate ISR lesions accurately [4].

However, blooming artifacts and beam-hardening artifacts induced by the metal stent affect the diagnostic performance. Model-based iterative reconstruction can help to improve diagnostic performance for detecting in-stent restenosis on coronary CTA images [5]. In addition, dual-energy CT acquisitions with virtual monoenergetic images can decrease beam-hardening artifacts caused by coronary stents and is increasingly clinically available [6]. Coronary stent subtraction CT imaging provides better diagnostic performance than conventional CCTA in the evaluation of in-stent restenosis by subtracting pre-contrast images from post-contrast images [7]. With the development of dual-energy technology, subtraction between conventional images, VNC (virtual non-enhancement) images, and different monoenergetic images may provide higher diagnostic performance without misregistration artifacts [8].

Diabetes, characteristic of stenosis lesions, number of and characteristic of stents, hereditary factors are the risk factors of ISR. Quantitative markers such as remodeling index, lesion length, and noncalcified plaque volumes derived from CCTA performed prior to percutaneous coronary intervention may have incremental predictive value for ISR [9].

Myocardial CT perfusion (CTP) is effective in the assessment of myocardial ischemia. For those suspected ISR, CTP and combined coronary CTA + CTP were able to improve the diagnostic performance of coronary CTA alone [10]. Another functional CT technology, FFR_{CT}, is not suitable for stent evaluation.

Cardiac CT examination plays an important role in predicting and detecting ISR.

3.4 Key Points

- ISR was identified by a darker area within the in-stent lumen, with >50% diameter stenosis. The presenting symptoms of ISR including stable angina, unstable angina, or myocardial infarction.
- With the development of CT imaging technologies, coronary CTA and myocardial CT perfusion have become increasingly used for detecting in-stent restenosis (ISR) during the follow-ups.

References

1. Mehran R, Dangas G, Abizaid AS, Mintz GS, Lansky AJ, Satler LF, et al. Angiographic patterns of in-stent restenosis: classification and implications for long-term outcome. Circulation. 1999;100(18):1872–8. https://doi.org/10.1161/01.cir.100.18.1872.

2. Sun Z, Almutairi AM. Diagnostic accuracy of 64 multislice CT angiography in the assessment of coronary in-stent restenosis: a meta-analysis. Eur J Radiol. 2010;73(2):266–73. https://doi.org/10.1016/j.ejrad.2008.10.025.

3. Magalhaes MA, Minha S, Chen F, Torguson R, Omar AF, Loh JP, et al. Clinical presentation and outcomes of coronary in-stent restenosis across 3-stent generations. Circ Cardiovasc Interv. 2014;7(6):768–76. https://doi.org/10.1161/circinterventions.114.001341.

4. Dai T, Wang JR, Hu PF. Diagnostic performance of computed tomography angiography in the detection of coronary artery in-stent restenosis: evidence from an updated meta-analysis. Eur Radiol. 2018;28(4):1373–82. https://doi.org/10.1007/s00330-017-5097-0.

5. Tatsugami F, Higaki T, Sakane H, Nakamura Y, Iida M, Baba Y, et al. Diagnostic accuracy of in-stent restenosis using model-based iterative reconstruction at coronary CT angiography: initial experience. Br J Radiol. 2018;91(1082):20170598. https://doi.org/10.1259/bjr.20170598.

6. Hickethier T, Baessler B, Kroeger JR, Doerner J, Pahn G, Maintz D, et al. Monoenergetic reconstructions for imaging of coronary artery stents using spectral detector CT: in-vitro experience and comparison to conventional images. J Cardiovasc Comput Tomogr. 2017;11(1):33–9. https://doi.org/10.1016/j.jcct.2016.12.005.

7. Fuchs A, Kuhl JT, Chen MY, Helqvist S, Razeto M, Arakita K, et al. Feasibility of coronary calcium and stent image subtraction using 320-detector row CT angiography. J Cardiovasc Comput Tomogr. 2015;9(5):393–8. https://doi.org/10.1016/j.jcct.2015.03.016.

8. Qin L, Gu S, Chen C, Zhang H, Zhu Z, Chen X, et al. Initial exploration of coronary stent image subtraction using dual-layer spectral CT. Eur Radiol. 2019;29(8):4239–48. https://doi.org/10.1007/s00330-018-5990-1.

9. Tesche C, De Cecco CN, Vliegenthart R, Duguay TM, Stubenrauch AC, Rosenberg RD, et al. Coronary CT angiography-derived quantitative markers for predicting in-stent restenosis. J Cardiovasc Comput Tomogr. 2016;10(5):377–83. https://doi.org/10.1016/j.jcct.2016.07.005.

10. Andreini D, Mushtaq S, Pontone G, Conte E, Collet C, Sonck J, et al. CT perfusion versus coronary CT angiography in patients with suspected in-stent restenosis or CAD progression. JACC Cardiovasc Imaging. 2019;13(3):732–42. https://doi.org/10.1016/j.jcmg.2019.05.031.

Dual-Energy Evaluation of High Calcium Score (>400) Coronary Artery

4

Peijun Liu, Yining Wang, and Zheng-yu Jin

Abstract

Coronary computed tomography angiography (CCTA) is widely used as a noninvasive cardiovascular imaging modality that allows visualization of both calcified and noncalcified atherosclerotic plaques and exclusion of coronary luminal stenoses with high diagnostic performance. However, high (>400) coronary artery calcium score (CACS) may increase the false-positive rate and decease diagnostic accuracy due to beam-hardening artifacts resulting from heavily calcified plaques. For patients with high CACS cannot be reliably evaluated with CCTA and invasive coronary angiography (ICA) is frequently recommended in routine clinical practice. Recently, dual-energy CT (DECT) has been introduced to reduce beam-hardening artifacts and improve the diagnostic performance of CCTA in patients with severe coronary calcification. In this chapter, we will investigate the implication of CACS and further discuss the application of DECT in patients with CACS.

4.1 Case of High Calcium Score (>400) Coronary Artery

4.1.1 History

A 52-year-old male patient felt sudden chest pain in the night, which travels to the left arm, shortness of breath, sweating, nausea, and vomiting 2 months ago. After taking medicine, his symptoms relieved. For further diagnosis, this patient came to our hospital and made a reservation for a cardiac CT examination due to suspected myocardial infarction.

4.1.1.1 Physical Examination
- Blood pressure: 103/73 mmHg
- Breathing rate: 15/min
- Heart rate: 67 bpm

4.1.1.2 Electrocardiograph
Reversed T wave, ST segment elevation.

4.1.1.3 Laboratory
Serum myocardial enzyme spectrum showed negative results.

P. Liu · Y. Wang · Z.-y. Jin (✉)
Department of Radiology, Peking Union Medical
College Hospital, Chinese Academy of Medical
Sciences and Peking Union Medical College,
Beijing, China
e-mail: jinzy@pumch.cn

© Springer Nature Singapore Pte Ltd. 2020
Z.-y. Jin et al. (eds.), *Cardiac CT*, https://doi.org/10.1007/978-981-15-5305-9_4

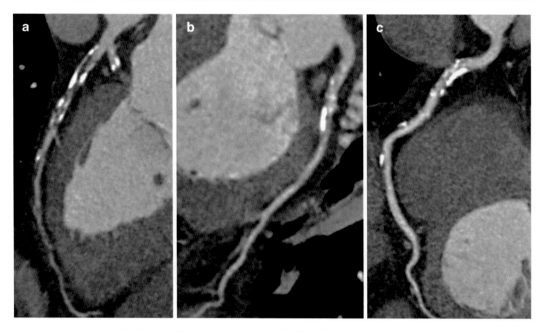

Fig. 4.1 Curved multi-planar (CPR) reconstructed images (**a**, left anterior descending [LAD]; **b**, left circumflex artery [LCX]; **c**, right coronary artery [RCA]) of the CCTA. There are multiple calcified plaque and mixed plaque in the three coronary arteries

4.1.2   Imaging Examination

4.1.2.1 CT Images
CCTA image was obtained from DECT to evaluate plaque and coronary lumen (Figs. 4.1 and 4.2)

4.1.2.2 Conventional Coronary
         Angiography (Fig. 4.3)

4.1.3   Imaging Findings
         and Diagnosis

The CCTA image results showed multiple mixed plaque in LAD, in which severe stenosis in the proximal and middle segment and moderate stenosis in the distal segment. There were multiple mixed plaques in the proximal–middle segments of LCX leading to severe stenosis. Mild-moderate stenosis exists in the middle segment resulting

from multiple mixed plaques of RCA. High monoenergetic imaging from DECT can decrease effectively calcified blooming artifact. The invasive coronary angiography images confirmed multiple stenosis in three coronary arteries.

4.1.4   Management

- Coronary artery bypass grafting operation
- Conventional medical therapy for coronary artery disease (CAD)

4.2   Discussion

Coronary artery calcium (CAC) is a highly specific feature of coronary atherosclerosis in CAD. The prevalence of CAC continues to increase with growing age, and men have higher

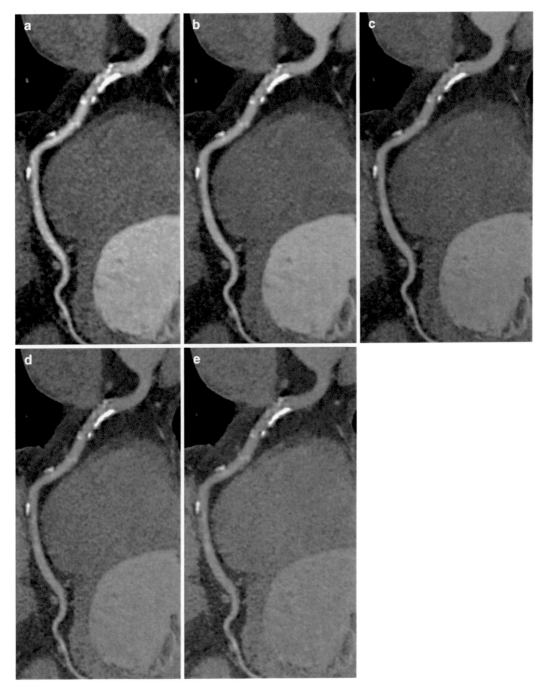

Fig. 4.2 Different monoenergetic image [(**a**) conventional CT image; (**b**) 80 keV monoenergetic image; (**c**) 100 keV monoenergetic image; (**d**) 120 keV monoenergetic image; (**e**) 150 keV monoenergetic image] were obtained from DECT. High monoenergetic image can reduce calcium blooming artifact

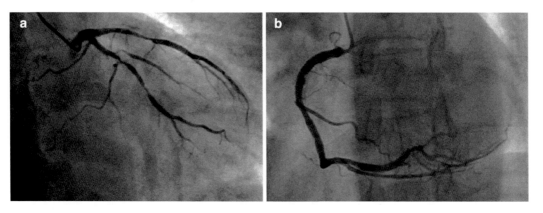

Fig. 4.3 Percutaneous coronary intervention (PCI) results. Invasive coronary angiography image for LAD (**a**), LCX (**a**) and RCA (**b**), confirmed multiple stenosis in three coronary arteries

calcium levels than women [1]. In addition, patients with high risk factors, such as diabetes mellitus, dyslipidemia, and hypertension, are more susceptible to CAC. The calcium score proposed by Agatston et al. remains the most widely accepted technique for predicting major adverse cardiovascular events and it is determined by the product of the total size and density of the calcified plaque deposited in the coronary artery tree [2]. Standardized categories for CACS include scores of 0 with the absence of calcified plaque, 1 to 10 with minimal plaque, 11 to 100 with mild plaque, 101 to 400 with moderate plaque, and >400 with severe plaque. And CACS >400 indicates significant prognostic implications in specific patient groups [3]. Other techniques for the measurement of coronary artery calcium are volume score and mass score [4].

Intravascular ultrasound (IVUS) has high diagnostic performance in identifying and characterizing plaque composition [5]. According to the range of calcified lesion detected by IVUS, CAC is divided into four classes: Class I with 0°–90° calcification, Class II with 91°–180° calcification, Class III with181°–270° calcification, and Class IV >270° calcification [3].

Optical coherence tomography (OCT) is also an intravascular imaging modality that enables providing cross-sectional images of tissue and has high sensitivity and specificity to identify atherosclerotic plaques [6]. Moreover, optical coherence tomography can be used to assess the thickness and volume of calcified plaque.

4.3 Current Technical Status and Applications of CT

DECT is a novel technology that allows the acquisition of two different datasets from two different X-ray spectra energies. Current techniques for DECT are divided into source-based and detector-based technique [7]. Source-based DECT includes dual-source scanner (two X-ray source–detector systems), rapid kVp switching scanner (a single X-ray source–detector system), dual-spin scanner (a single X-ray source and a single detector layer), and twin-beam scanner (X-ray beam is split into two energy spectra by pre-filtration). Detector-based DECT includes dual-layer detector and photon counting scanner. These techniques not only provide new clinical application for cardiac CT, but also overcome some disadvantages which exist in conventional CT.

Virtual monoenergetic imaging (VMI) generated from DECT reconstruction is analogous to imaging with a monoenergetic beam at single kiloelectron voltage (keV). Although calcium blooming artifact from coronary calcified plaque can lead to overestimate lumen stenosis at conventional CT, it is reduced at DECT by using high monoenergetic imaging. There are some evidences that calcium blooming effectively decreases at higher monoenergetic levels [8, 9]. Moreover, the use of monochromatic reconstructions improved the overall accuracy of coronary stenosis assessment using ICA as a standard of reference [10].

Calcium subtraction imaging can be obtained at conventional CT, but this technique will increase image misregistration risk and radiation dose [11]. In contrast, DECT has the ability to differentiate intravascular calcium from iodine contrast medium based on its material decomposition during image acquisition. Consequently, virtual calcium subtracted images derived from DECT were generated using dedicated subtraction algorithms. The study of De Santis D et al. demonstrated a prototype calcium subtraction algorithm from DECT that can improve coronary lumen assessment and increase diagnostic confidence in patients with heavy calcified coronary artery [12].

Virtual non-contrast (VNC) imaging is characterized by iodine elimination from CT angiographic imaging. Compared with true non-contrast imaging, VNC imaging can be obtained at one acquisition and thereby reduce radiation dose. Moreover, this technique can be used to differentiate contrast medium and other non-iodine material, such as calcified plaque and mental implanted material. VNC imaging can be used for CACS analysis. CACS from VNC imaging has excellent correlations compared with those from true non-contrast imaging [13, 14].

DECT provides multiple possibilities for calcified plaque analysis by different reconstruction algorithms, which are beneficial to disease diagnosis and clinical management.

4.4 Key Points

- CACS is a reliable technique for cardiac events risk evaluation.
- High keV monoenergetic imaging can decrease calcium blooming artifact.
- Calcium subtraction imaging and VNC imaging can reduce radiation dose.

References

1. McClelland RL, Chung H, Detrano R, Post W, Kronmal RA. Distribution of coronary artery calcium by race, gender, and age: results from the multi-ethnic study of atherosclerosis (MESA). Circulation. 2006;113(1):30–7. https://doi.org/10.1161/circulationaha.105.580696.
2. Agatston AS, Janowitz WR, Hildner FJ, Zusmer NR, Viamonte M, Detrano R. Quantification of coronary artery calcium using ultrafast computed tomography. J Am Coll Cardiol. 1990;15(4):827–32. https://doi.org/10.1016/0735-1097(90)90282-t.
3. Liu W, Zhang Y, Yu CM, Ji QW, Cai M, Zhao YX, et al. Current understanding of coronary artery calcification. J Geriatr Cardiol. 2015;12(6):668–75. https://doi.org/10.11909/j.issn.1671-5411.2015.06.012.
4. Alluri K, Joshi PH, Henry TS, Blumenthal RS, Nasir K, Blaha MJ. Scoring of coronary artery calcium scans: history, assumptions, current limitations, and future directions. Atherosclerosis. 2015;239(1):109–17. https://doi.org/10.1016/j.atherosclerosis.2014.12.040.
5. Nair A, Kuban BD, Tuzcu EM, Schoenhagen P, Nissen SE, Vince DG. Coronary plaque classification with intravascular ultrasound radiofrequency data analysis. Circulation. 2002;106(17):2200–6. https://doi.org/10.1161/01.cir.0000035654.18341.5e.
6. Yabushita H, Bouma BE, Houser SL, Aretz HT, Jang IK, Schlendorf KH, et al. Characterization of human atherosclerosis by optical coherence tomography. Circulation. 2002;106(13):1640–5. https://doi.org/10.1161/01.cir.0000029927.92825.f6.
7. Kalisz K, Halliburton S, Abbara S, Leipsic JA, Albrecht MH, Schoepf UJ, et al. Update on cardiovascular applications of multienergy CT. Radiographics. 2017;37(7):1955–74. https://doi.org/10.1148/rg.2017170100.
8. Van Hedent S, Hokamp NG, Kessner R, Gilkeson R, Ros PR, Gupta A. Effect of virtual monoenergetic images from spectral detector computed tomography on coronary calcium blooming. J Comput Assist Tomogr. 2018;42(6):912–8. https://doi.org/10.1097/RCT.0000000000000811.
9. Yu L, Leng S, McCollough CH. Dual-energy CT-based monochromatic imaging. AJR Am J Roentgenol. 2012;199(5 Suppl):S9–s15. https://doi.org/10.2214/ajr.12.9121.
10. Stehli J, Clerc OF, Fuchs TA, Possner M, Gräni C, Benz DC, et al. Impact of monochromatic coronary computed tomography angiography from single-source dual-energy CT on coronary stenosis quantification. J Cardiovasc Comput Tomogr. 2016;10(2):135–40. https://doi.org/10.1016/j.jcct.2015.12.008.
11. De Santis D, Eid M, De Cecco CN, Jacobs BE, Albrecht MH, Varga-Szemes A, et al. Dual-energy computed tomography in cardiothoracic vascular imaging. Radiol Clin N Am. 2018;56(4):521–34. https://doi.org/10.1016/j.rcl.2018.03.010.

12. De Santis D, Jin KN, Schoepf UJ, Grant KL, De Cecco CN, Nance JW, et al. Heavily calcified coronary arteries: advanced calcium subtraction improves luminal visualization and diagnostic confidence in dual-energy coronary computed tomography angiography. Investig Radiol. 2018;53(2):103–9. https://doi.org/10.1097/rli.0000000000000416.

13. Song I, Yi JG, Park JH, Kim SM, Lee KS, Chung MJ. Virtual non-contrast CT using dual-energy spectral CT: feasibility of coronary artery calcium scoring. Korean J Radiol. 2016;17(3):321–9. https://doi.org/10.3348/kjr.2016.17.3.321.

14. Schwarz F, Nance JW, Ruzsics B, Bastarrika G, Sterzik A, Schoepf UJ. Quantification of coronary artery calcium on the basis of dual-energy coronary CT angiography. Radiology. 2012;264(3):700–7. https://doi.org/10.1148/radiol.12112455.

Dual-Energy Evaluation of Coronary Artery Stent

5

Cheng Xu and Yining Wang

Abstract

Coronary artery stenting has been an important therapeutic procedure for patients with coronary artery stenosis and the number of patients who received stenting is increasing. As a noninvasive method, coronary computed tomography angiography (CTA) has become increasingly used during the follow-up. However, beam-hardening artifacts, appearing as dark areas adjacent to metal stents, limit the diagnostic performance of cardiac CT, especially when the stent diameter is <3 mm. Recently, with the rapid technologic advances, dual-energy CT (DECT) has been applied in many clinical areas. With dual-energy CT, attenuation data from different energies are used to characterize materials, virtual monoenergetic images (VMI) and stent subtraction images can be used to improve the diagnostic performance of stent evaluation. In this chapter, based on a case, we will discuss the assessment of coronary stent by dual-energy CT imaging, and further possibly promising role of CT technology in coronary stent evaluation.

C. Xu · Y. Wang (✉)
Department of Radiology, Peking Union Medical College Hospital, Chinese Academy of Medical Sciences and Peking Union Medical College, Beijing, China
e-mail: wangyining@pumch.cn

5.1 Case of Coronary Stent

5.1.1 History

A 53-year-old male patient felt chest distress and chest pain lasting for an hour several days ago. He had a history of PCI a year ago and the stent was implanted in the proximal segment of left anterior descending artery (LAD). He was appointed to coronary CTA for suspected in-stent restenosis or coronary artery disease (CAD) progression.

Physical Examination
- Blood pressure: 123/82 mmHg; Breathing rate: 18/min
- Heart rate: 64 bpm without arrhythmia

Electrocardiograph
- Standard 12-lead electrocardiograph (ECG) revealed no abnormality.

Laboratory
- Serum myocardial enzyme spectrum showed negative results.

5.1.2 Imaging Examination

CT Images
Coronary CT angiography (CTA) was performed on dual-layer detector CT (Figs. 5.1, 5.2, and 5.3).

© Springer Nature Singapore Pte Ltd. 2020
Z.-y. Jin et al. (eds.), *Cardiac CT*, https://doi.org/10.1007/978-981-15-5305-9_5

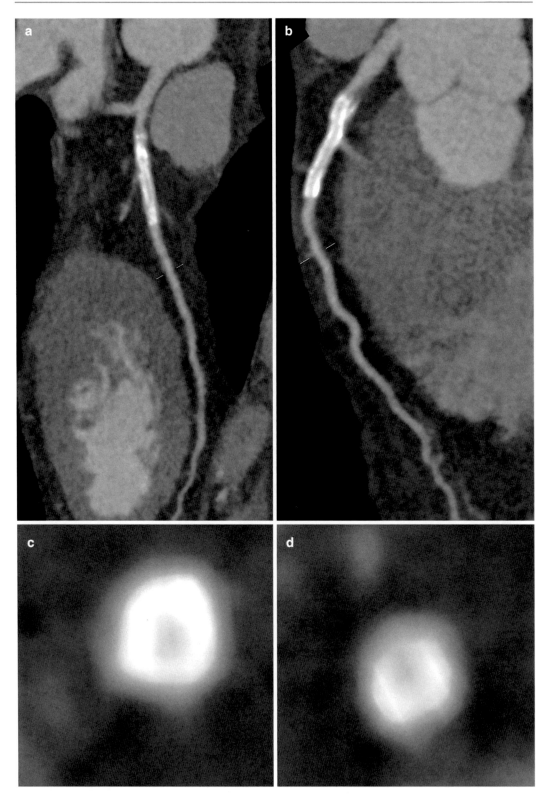

Fig. 5.1 Coronary CTA B26f. Curved multi-planar (CPR) reconstructed images (**a** and **b**, left anterior descending artery [LAD]) and transverse section of the stent (**c** and **d**). The in-stent lumen patency of proximal LAD was hard to diagnose due to beam-hardening artifact

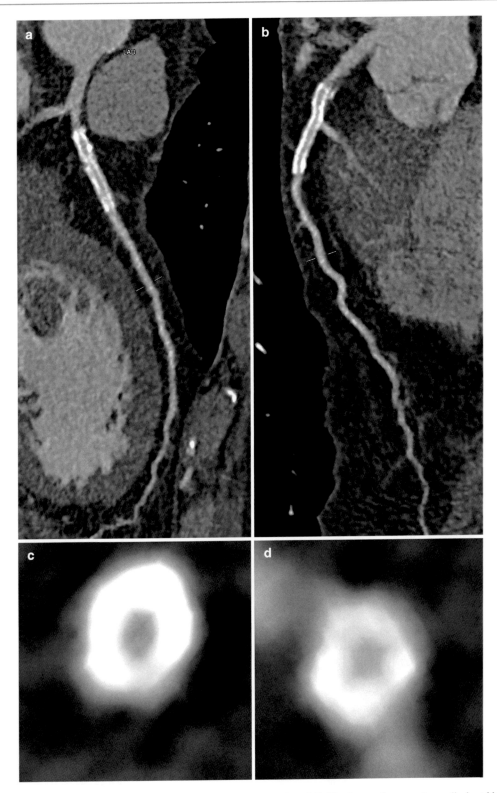

Fig. 5.2 Coronary CTA B46f. Curved multi-planar (CPR) reconstructed images (**a** and **b**, left anterior descending artery [LAD]) and transverse section of the stent (**c** and **d**). The in-stent lumen patency displayed better than that on B26f

Conventional   Coronary   Angiography
(Fig. 5.4)

5.1.3   Imaging Findings and Diagnosis

The coronary CTA images results showed the in-stent lumen patency of LAD was hard to diagnose because of beam-hardening artifacts (B26f).

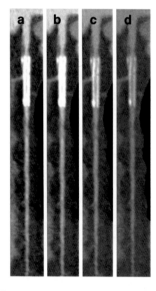

Fig. 5.3 Conventional polychromatic images (**a**), mono 70 keV (**b**), mono 90 keV (**c**) and mono 100 keV (**d**) of LAD. Higher energy level can minimize the beam-hardening artifact and there is no ISR

The curved multiplanar reconstruction of LAD on sharp convolution kernel (B46f) displayed the in-stent lumen of LAD better; there was no in-stent restenosis but there were noncalcified plaques in the proximal and middle segment of LAD, resulting in mild lumen stenosis. On virtual monoenergetic images, the window level and window width were set at 90 and 750, respectively; it was obvious that 100 keV image displays the stent better than conventional images and there was no ISR. The invasive coronary angiography images confirmed that there was no ISR but moderate stenosis in middle LAD, which may contribute to the symptoms.

5.1.4   Management

- Conventional medical therapy for CAD and clinical follow-up

5.2   Discussion

Coronary artery stenting has been widely introduced into clinical practice. Patients who undergo PCI experience a reduction or disappearance of symptoms. However, caused by intimal hyperplasia, in-stent restenosis is one of the main limitations of stent placement. Usually, invasive coronary angiography is performed when ISR is

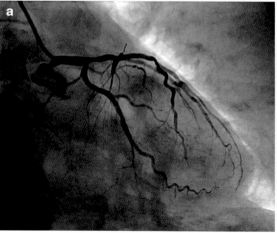
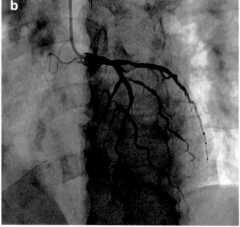

Fig. 5.4 Invasive coronary angiography image for LAD (**a** and **b**). The result show there was no in-stent restenosis in LAD but 70% stenosis in middle LAD

clinically suspected. Accurate evaluation of stents has always been a challenge on coronary CTA. Recently, with the development of dual-energy CT, the in-lumen visibility of small stents and the diagnostic performance of coronary CTA have been improved. On coronary CTA, stent patency can be visually evaluated. If ISR happens, a darker area between the stent and the enhanced lumen can be found. Image quality can be quantified by image noise, visible lumen diameter, and in-stent attenuation difference.

5.3 Current Technical Status and Applications of CT

In order to acquire the dual-energy data set, various technical approaches have been developed, including two temporally sequential scans, rapid switching of X-ray tube potential, multilayer detector, dual X-ray sources, and photon-counting detectors [1]. By these approaches, image sets can be created in the projection domain or in the image domain. DECT allows the creation of virtual monoenergetic reconstructions in which attenuation data approximate data that would be obtained with a mono-energy X-ray beam. Images can be created from 40 to 200 keV. VMI reconstructions at low energy allow for contrast dose reduction and image noise reduction while reconstructions at a high energy level can minimize the beam-hardening artifact [2, 3]. The visible lumen diameter, in-stent attenuation difference, image quality of VMI are better than conventional images [4].

Coronary stent subtraction CT imaging is another way to improve the diagnostic performance of coronary CTA. By subtracting non-contrast images from contrast-enhanced images, stents can be eliminated. Misregistration artifacts is a major limitation of stent subtraction CT imaging due to patient movement or changing HR [5]. With the development of dual-energy

technology, iodine data can be subtracted from contrast-enhanced images to create virtual non-enhanced images, subtraction between virtual non-enhancement images and monochromatic or mixed-energy images could yield equally improved in-stent lumen visibility and diagnostic accuracy without misregistration artifact.

DECT with various reconstruction images help in the accurate evaluation of stents.

5.4 Key Points

- In-stent restenosis is one of the main limitations of PCI treatment.
- DECT with virtual monoenergetic images and stent subtraction images help to evaluate in-stent lumen more accurately in CTA.

References

1. McCollough CH, Leng S, Yu L, Fletcher JG. Dual- and multi-energy CT: principles, technical approaches, and clinical applications. Radiology. 2015;276(3):637–53. https://doi.org/10.1148/radiol.2015142631.
2. Secchi F, De Cecco CN, Spearman JV, Silverman JR, Ebersberger U, Sardanelli F, et al. Monoenergetic extrapolation of cardiac dual energy CT for artifact reduction. Acta Radiol. 2015;56(4):413–8. https://doi.org/10.1177/0284185114527867.
3. Yu L, Leng S, McCollough CH. Dual-energy CT-based monochromatic imaging. AJR Am J Roentgenol. 2012;199(5 Suppl):S9–s15. https://doi.org/10.2214/ajr.12.9121.
4. Hickethier T, Baessler B, Kroeger JR, Doerner J, Pahn G, Maintz D, et al. Monoenergetic reconstructions for imaging of coronary artery stents using spectral detector CT: in-vitro experience and comparison to conventional images. J Cardiovasc Comput Tomogr. 2017;11(1):33–9. https://doi.org/10.1016/j.jcct.2016.12.005.
5. Fuchs A, Kuhl JT, Chen MY, Helqvist S, Razeto M, Arakita K, et al. Feasibility of coronary calcium and stent image subtraction using 320-detector row CT angiography. J Cardiovasc Comput Tomogr. 2015;9(5):393–8. https://doi.org/10.1016/j.jcct.2015.03.016.

Coronary Artery Bypass Grafting

6

Jia Liu and Jianxing Qiu

Abstract

Coronary artery bypass grafting (CABG) surgery is the standard treatment method of advanced coronary artery disease. In the past, invasive coronary angiography was used to assess the status of the grafts and check out if the graft was occluded. Recently, multidetector computed tomography (CT) with electrocardiographic (ECG) gating has become an important diagnostic tool for the evaluation of CABGs in postoperative settings. In this chapter, based on a case of a patient after a CABG surgery, we will discuss the coronary CT angiography (CCTA) imaging evaluation of CABGs.

6.1 Case of CABG

6.1.1 History

A 74-year-old male patient had a CABG surgery because of progressive exertional chest pain 16 years ago. His chest pain was aggravated in 3 months, which cannot be relieved by oral nitroglycerin and appointed to CCTA for further evaluation.

J. Liu · J. Qiu (✉)
Radiology Department, Peking University First Hospital, Beijing, China

6.1.1.1 Physical Examination
- Blood pressure: 148/84 mmHg
- Breathing rate: 18/min
- Heart rate: 70 bpm without arrhythmia

6.1.1.2 ECG
Standard 12-lead ECG revealed no obvious ST segment changes, but flat T wave on several leads.

6.1.1.3 Laboratory
Serum myocardial enzyme spectrum showed negative results.

6.1.2 Imaging Examination
(Figs. 6.1, 6.2, 6.3, and 6.4)

6.1.3 Imaging Findings

The patient received two left saphenous vein grafts (SVGs), a right radial artery and a left internal mammary artery (IMA) graft (Fig. 6.1). Curved multi-planar reconstructed (CPR) images showed there were mixed plaques in the three coronary arteries, and resulted in severe lumen stenosis (Fig. 6.2). No significant stenosis has been shown in the left IMA graft and distal segment of LAD. Note the smaller diameter of the arterial graft compared with that of the venous graft, and there are metal clips around the IMA

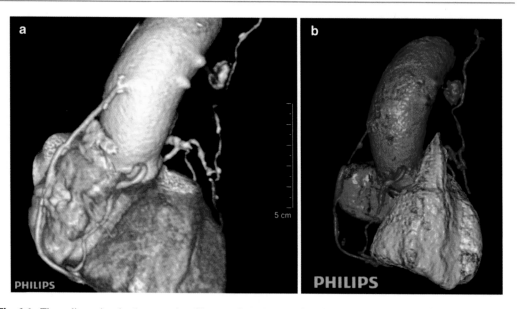

Fig. 6.1 Three-dimensional volume-rendered images show there are four CABGs. The patient received two left SVGs, a right radial artery graft and a left IMA graft. Images in (**a**) and (**b**) were reconstructed in different colors

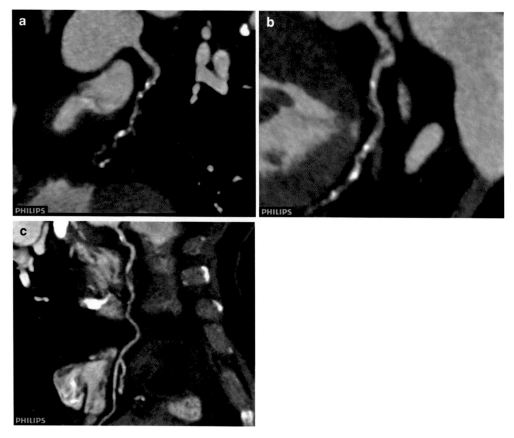

Fig. 6.2 CPR reconstructed images (**a**, left anterior descending [LAD] branch; **b**, left circumflex artery [LCX] and **c**, right coronary artery [RCA]) showed there were mixed plaques in the three coronary arteries, and resulted in severe lumen stenosis

graft. There is also a right radial artery attached to the posterior descending artery. The radial artery is smaller in caliber than the SVG and similar in size to the IMA graft. Maximum intensity projection image shows contrast material within only a short proximal segment of an SVG representing complete occlusion of the SVG (Fig. 6.3). Multidetector CT images show an SVG with an aneurysmal dilatation with a diameter of 1.4 cm, and secondary thrombosis with low density resulting in complete occlusion, which was near the ascending aorta, and there was no contrast material within the distal segment of the SVG (Fig. 6.4).

6.1.4   Management

- He took a percutaneous transluminal coronary intervention (PCI) operation and put a stent in LAD.
- Conventional medical therapy for CAD and outpatient follow-up observations.

6.2   Discussion

The various conduits used for CABG surgery may be divided into venous and arterial grafts. Venous grafts have shown a tendency to develop partial

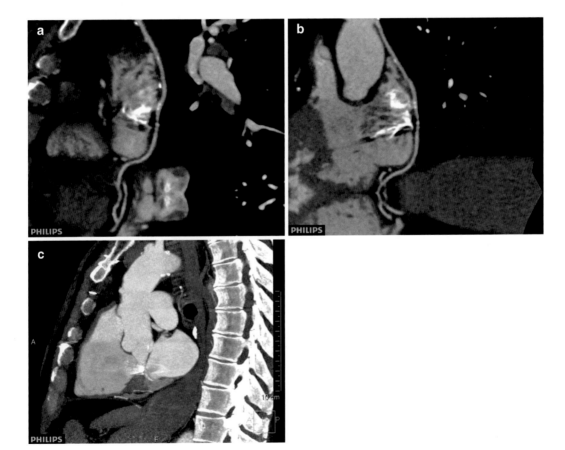

Fig. 6.3 (**a**) CPR reconstructed image shows no significant stenosis has been shown in the left IMA graft and distal segment of LAD. There are metal clips around the IMA graft. (**b**) CPR reconstructed image shows there is a right radial artery, which is attached to the posterior descending artery. No significant stenosis has been shown in the right radial artery graft. (**c**) Maximum intensity projection image shows contrast material within only a short proximal segment of an SVG representing complete occlusion of the SVG

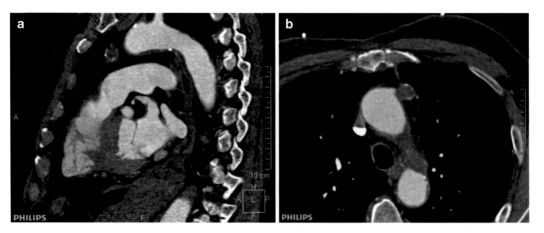

Fig. 6.4 Axial (**a**) and sagittal (**b**) multidetector CT images show an SVG with an aneurysmal dilatation and secondary thrombosis, which was near the ascending aorta

or complete occlusions with time. Arterial grafts have demonstrated relative resistance to plaque formation and obstruction, which are more limited in their availability and ease of procurement compared with venous grafts. Therefore, SVGs remain the most commonly used conduits [1].

SVGs are grafted from the anterior aspect of the ascending aorta to the distal coronary artery beyond the obstructive coronary lesion. At postoperative multidetector CT, the proximal segment of a graft is typically better visualized than its distal segment. Venous bypass grafts are typically larger in diameter than the native large epicardial coronary arteries, and they are less subjected to cardiac motion. Typically, the right IMA is left in place and the left IMA is used as the graft. Its origin at the subclavian artery remains intact and the distal end is connected to the target vessel, distal to the site of occlusion. CT evaluation is hampered by a relatively small diameter and metal clips around the IMA graft. Owing to the success of IMA grafts, other arterial bypass grafts are developed such as the radial artery, which is selected because of its ease of procurement from the forearm [1, 2].

Occlusion after the first month following the CABG surgery is primarily due to thrombosis, which results from exposure of the vein graft to systemic blood pressure and a process of arterialization. After surgery, progressive thickening of the media and neointimal formation form a foun-

dation for eventual atherosclerotic narrowing, which may ultimately lead to late graft occlusion. In contradistinction, IMA grafts are strikingly resistant to atheroma formation, which results in higher long-term patency rates than for SVGs. Late IMA graft failure more commonly occurs due to progressive atherosclerotic disease of the grafted native vessel distal to the anastomosis [1].

When an aneurysmal dilatation of a bypass graft exceeds 2 cm, it generally requires surgical correction. True aneurysms typically arise more than 5 years after surgery and occur in the body of the graft related to accelerated atherosclerosis. Pseudoaneurysms more commonly occur within 6 months after bypass, and earlier-onset cases may be related to tension at the anastomosis that leads to suture rupture or wound infection. However, the pathogenesis of later pseudoaneurysms most likely involves progressive atherosclerosis [1].

6.3 Current Technical Status and Applications of CT

Various imaging techniques are expected to overcome the limitations of standard coronary CT, which include beam-hardening artifacts, insufficient spatial and temporal resolution, and an inability to allow functional assessment of coronary stenosis. The use of a high-pitch dual-source helical scan, a step and shoot scan, and iterative reconstruction can further reduce radiation dose. High-definition CT can improve spatial resolution and diagnostic evaluation of small or peripheral coronary vessels and coronary stents. Dual-energy CT can improve contrast medium enhancement and reasonably reduce the contrast dose when combined with noise reduction with the use of iterative reconstruction. Dual-source CT and a motion correction algorithm can improve temporal resolution and reduce coronary motion artifacts. These new technologies have been recently applied to graft evaluation after bypass surgery [3, 4].

Patency of the CABG is often the most pressing clinical question in the evaluation of the CABG patient after surgery. The advancing technology of ECG gating multidetector CT now allows the radiologist to address this clinical concern in a rapid, convenient, and noninvasive manner. CTA is particularly effective in studying bypass grafts due to their large size, lower degree of calcifications, and decreased motion when compared to native vessels [5]. In addition, multidetector CT has the added advantage of simultaneous evaluation for alternate postoperative complications that may also manifest with chest pain and dyspnea. In order to minimize the risk of injury to a graft vessel during reentry, multidetector CT in preoperative planning before repeat CABG surgery is applied due to its improvements in spatial resolution and the ability to generate three-dimensional and multiplanar images. The role of multidetector CT evaluation of the CABG patient after surgery is likely to increase in the near future [1].

6.4 Key Points

- SVGs remain the most commonly used conduits. Venous grafts have demonstrated a tendency to develop partial or complete occlusions with time. Arterial grafts have shown relative resistance to plaque formation and obstruction.
- Recently, multidetector CT with ECG gating has become an important diagnostic tool for the evaluation of CABG in postoperative settings.

References

1. Frazier AA, Qureshi F, Read KM, et al. Coronary artery bypass grafts: assessment with multidetector CT in the early and late postoperative settings. Radiographics. 2005;25(4):881–96.
2. Schmermund A, Möhlenkamp S, Schlosser T, et al. Coronary angiography after revascularization. In: Budoff MJ, Shinbane JS, editors. Cardiac CT imaging: diagnosis of cardiovascular disease. Cham: Springer. p. 135–45.
3. Lazzaro DD, Crusco F. CT angio for the evaluation of graft patency. J Thorac Dis. 2017;9(4):283–8.
4. Machida H, Tanaka I, Fukui R, et al. Current and novel imaging techniques in coronary CT. Radiographics. 2015;35(4):991–1010.
5. Eisenberg C, Hulten E, Bittencourt MS, et al. Use of CT angiography among patients with prior coronary artery bypass grafting surgery. Cardiovascu Diagn Ther. 2017;7(1):102–5.

Borderline Lesion Evaluation: CT-FFR

7

Yan Yi, Jingwen Dai, and Yining Wang

Abstract

Fractional flow reserve (FFR) is an index defined as the ratio of maximum coronary blood flow distal to a stenosis lesion to normal maximum coronary blood flow in the same vessel in the hypothesis that the vessel is normal. FFR is considered as the gold standard in determining the severity of coronary artery stenosis and for guiding the decision-making to identify patients who will benefit from revascularization. FFR is usually obtained during invasive coronary angiography and required administration of adenosine. Fractional flow reserve derived from coronary computed tomography angiography (CT-FFR) allows the evaluation of the hemodynamic severity of coronary artery lesions in a noninvasive way and assessing the anatomic stenosis of a coronary artery with its functional effects. Now CT-FFR is considered as a powerful tool for the depiction of lesion-specific ischemia and has high diagnostic value. In this chapter, based on a case of coronary artery disease (CAD), we will discuss the CT-FFR in evaluating the anatomy and hemodynamics of coronary artery stenosis.

7.1 Case of CT-FFR

7.1.1 History

- A 72-year-old female patient has been feeling progressive exertional chest tightness for the past year.
- He appointed to coronary CT angiography for suspected CAD.

7.1.1.1 Physical Examination
- Blood pressure: 148/80 mmHg; Breathing rate: 18/min
- Heart rate: 70 bpm without arrhythmia

7.1.1.2 Laboratory
Thyroid hormone examination showed hyperthyroidism.

7.1.2 Imaging Examination

7.1.2.1 CT Images
A coronary CT angiography (CTA) was requested to evaluate the coronary artery and the coronary blood flow (Figs. 7.1 and 7.2).

Y. Yi · J. Dai · Y. Wang (✉)
Department of Radiology, Peking Union Medical College Hospital, Chinese Academy of Medical Sciences and Peking Union Medical College, Beijing, China
e-mail: wangyining@pumch.cn

© Springer Nature Singapore Pte Ltd. 2020
Z.-y. Jin et al. (eds.), *Cardiac CT*, https://doi.org/10.1007/978-981-15-5305-9_7

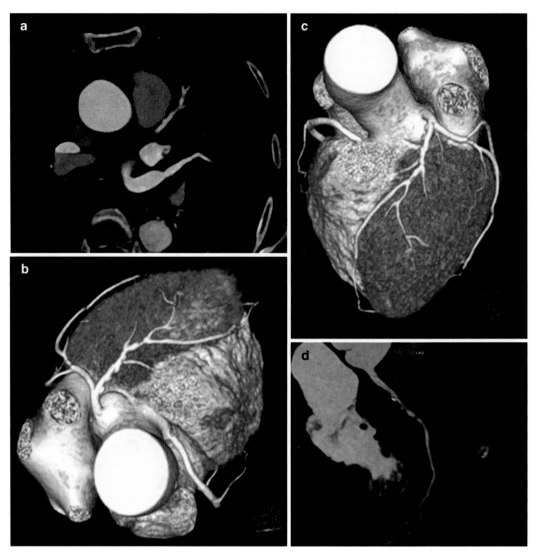

Fig. 7.1 Maximum intensity projection (MIP) image (**a**), curved multi-planar (CPR) reconstructed image (**d**) and volume rendering technique (VRT) image (**b–f**) of the coronary CTA showed a mixed plaque in the mid-segment of the left artery descending (LAD) and resulted in 70% stenosis

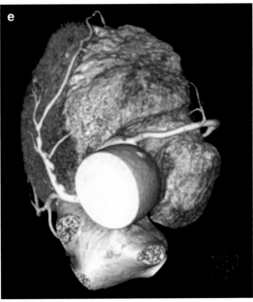
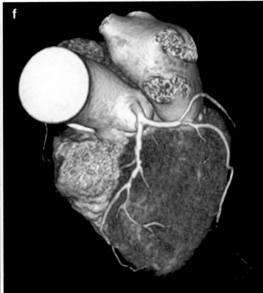

Fig. 7.1 (continued)

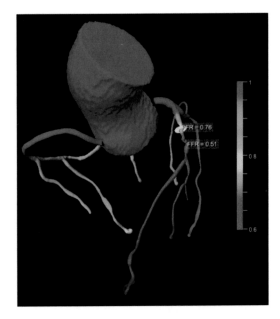

Fig. 7.2 CT-FFR analysis showed the proximal and distal value of the LAD stenosis was 0.76 and 0.51, respectively

7.1.2.2 Conventional Coronary Angiography and FFR (Fig. 7.3)

7.1.3 Imaging Findings and Diagnosis

The coronary CTA images showed there were mixed plaques in the middle segment of LAD and resulted in 70% luminal stenosis. No significant stenosis has been found in other coronary arteries. CT-FFR was calculated according to the CTA images. And the CT-FFR analysis showed the proximal and distal value of the LAD stenosis was 0.76 and 0.51, respectively. The invasive coronary angiography images conformed a significant stenosis in the middle segment of LAD and a distal FFR value of 0.60 indicating a hemodynamically significant stenosis (<0.80), which is consistent with CTA results.

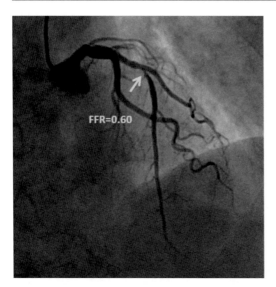

FFR=0.60

Fig. 7.3 Percutaneous transluminal coronary intervention (PCI) results. Invasive coronary angiography image for LAD showed a significant stenosis and the distal FFR value was 0.60

7.1.4 Management

- Coronary stent implantation in the middle segment of LAD.
- Conventional medical therapy for secondary prevention of CAD.
- Out-patient follow-up observations for CAD.

7.2 Discussion

Coronary computed tomography angiography (CCTA) is one of the first choice methods for noninvasive evaluation of coronary anatomy. It has been proved to have high sensitivity and negative predictive value and turned out to be an excellent tool for ruling out coronary artery stenosis. Traditional CCTA is an anatomic imaging modality incapable to evaluate the hemodynamic parameter of coronary stenosis lesions. However, anatomical coronary stenosis severity does not always correlate well with the hemodynamic severity evaluated by invasive FFR.

An array of studies have demonstrated that the FFR-guided PCI can alleviate symptoms and improve prognosis [1, 2]. But the clinical application as an initial choice in evaluating coronary stenosis

has been limited owing to its invasive nature. FFR derived from CCTA images has become a novel noninvasive modality to evaluate the functional severity of CAD. CT-FFR is calculated by computational flow modeling using the same images used for evaluating coronary arteries without the administration of adenosine. Extra image acquisition, radiation exposure, or stress during CCTA scanning are not necessary for calculating CT-FFR.

Coronary lesions with FFR < 0.75 are considered as hemodynamic significant, while stenosis with FFR > 0.80 is not considered to be associated with ischemia. And the diagnostic performance of CT-FFR in assessing lesion-specific ischemia in CAD patients has been investigated in many clinical trials and the results demonstrated that among stable CAD patients CT-FFR using FFR as the reference standard has excellent diagnostic performance, with high sensitivity in detecting anatomic stenosis of coronary artery and high specificity for evaluating ischemia lesions, which will increase the clinical use of CTA in the assessment and management of CAD in the future [3, 4].

7.3 Current Technical Status and Applications of CT-FFR

CT-FFR is a novel noninvasive modality to evaluate the coronary stenosis both anatomically and hemodynamically and for accurate detection of ischemia causing coronary lesions. It is calculated through computational fluid dynamics using typically acquired coronary CTA images without additional imaging or adenosine.

Calculation of CT-FFR needs several steps. First, patient-specific anatomic models from coronary CTA need to be established and the total and vessel-specific baseline coronary artery flow should be quantified in the hypothesis that the supplying artery is normal. Second, the baseline myocardial microcirculatory resistance needs to be determined and also the quantification of the changes in coronary resistance with hyperemia. And then the coronary flow, pressure, and velocity at rest and hyperemia will be calculated by the application of computational fluid dynamics methods [5, 6].

Three prospective, multicenter clinical trials using blinded core laboratory controls have been conducted to evaluate the diagnostic performance of CT-FFR using measured FFR as the reference standard, the DISCOVER-FLOW [7], DeFACTO [8], and NXT [9]. The results demonstrated that CT-FFR significantly improved the diagnostic accuracy in detecting ischemia compared with coronary CTA. The per-vessel accuracy and specificity to detect stenosis that was responsible for myocardial ischemia were significantly higher for CT-FFR than for coronary CTA [7–9]. For the prognosis in CAD patients, a previous study showed there was a trend toward more patients with a CT-FFR ≤ 0.80 experiencing major adverse cardiovascular events at 12 months compared with the patients with a CT-FFR > 0.80 [10].

CT-FFR has become a powerful and promising tool for evaluating coronary stenosis. It is the only noninvasive imaging tool for the detection of lesion-specific ischemia, and many studies have demonstrated its good diagnostic performance and allows the prediction of outcome in CAD patients.

7.4 Key Points

- CT-FFR is a powerful tool in evaluating the coronary stenosis severity both anatomically and functionally, and showed excellent diagnostic and prognostic value.

References

1. De Bruyne B, Fearon WF, Pijls NH, et al. Fractional flow reserve-guided PCI for stable coronary artery disease. N Engl J Med. 2014;371:1208–17.
2. De Bruyne B, Pijls NH, Kalesan B, et al. Fractional flow reserve-guided PCI versus medical therapy in stable coronary disease. N Engl J Med. 2012;367:991–1001.
3. Pijls NH, Fearon WF, Tonino PA, et al. Fractional flow reserve versus angiography for guiding percutaneous coronary intervention in patients with multivessel coronary artery disease: 2-year follow-up of the FAME (fractional flow reserve versus angiography for multivessel evaluation) study. J Am Coll Cardiol. 2010;56:177–84.
4. Tonino PA, De Bruyne B, Pijls NH, et al. Fractional flow reserve versus angiography for guiding percutaneous coronary intervention. N Engl J Med. 2009;360:213–24.
5. Taylor CA, Fonte TA, Min JK, et al. Computational fluid dynamics applied to cardiac computed tomography for noninvasive quantification of fractional flow reserve: scientific basis. J Am Coll Cardiol. 2013;61:2233–41.
6. Kim HJ, Vignon-Clementel IE, Coogan JS, et al. Patient specific modeling of blood flow and pressure in human coronary arteries. Ann Biomed Eng. 2010;38:3195–209.
7. Koo BK, Erglis A, Doh JH, et al. Diagnosis of ischemia-causing coronary stenoses by noninvasive fractional flow reserve computed from coronary computed tomographic angiograms. Results from the prospective multicenter DISCOVER-FLOW (diagnosis of ischemia-causing stenoses obtained via noninvasive fractional flow reserve) study. J Am Coll Cardiol. 2011;58:1989–97. This was the first pioneer study demonstrating feasibility of coronary FFRCT testing
8. Min JK, Leipsic J, Pencina MJ, et al. Diagnostic accuracy of fractional flow reserve from anatomic CT angiography. JAMA. 2012;308:1237–45.
9. Nørgaard BL, Leipsic J, Gaur S, et al. Diagnostic performance of noninvasive fractional flow reserve derived from coronary computed tomography angiography in suspected coronary artery disease: the NXT trial. J Am Coll Cardiol. 2014;63:1145–55.
10. Lu MT, Ferencik M, Roberts RC, et al. Noninvasive FFR derived from coronary CT angiography: management and outcomes in the PROMISE trial. JACC Cardiovasc Imag. 2017;10(11):1350–8.

Takayasu's Arteritis

8

Jian Cao, Yining Wang, and Zheng-yu Jin

Abstract

Takayasu's arteritis (TAK) is classified as a large-vessel vasculitis because it primarily affects the aorta and its primary branches. The thickening and fibrosis of the whole wall of the artery were diffuse or irregular, which resulted in the stenosis and occlusion of the artery. The patient initially presented with systemic symptoms, followed by vascular injury. 80–90% of the cases are female, and the age of onset is usually between 10 and 40 years. Imaging examination is very important for the diagnosis of TAK and assessment of the extent of vascular lesions. Patients suspected of TAK should be evaluated by CTA or MRA.

8.1 Case of TAK

8.1.1 History

- A 23-year-old woman complained of fever with cough for more than 1 year.
- She had cough with white phlegm, intermittent hemoptysis with chest pain and had low fever in the evening; the body temperature was about 37.5 °C.
- No improvement after anti-inflammatory treatment, and weight loss of about 5 kg in recent 6 months.

8.1.1.1 Physical Examination
- Blood pressure: 125/74 mmHg; Breathing rate: 20/min
- Heart rate: 92 bpm without arrhythmia

8.1.1.2 Electrocardiograph
Standard 12-lead electrocardiograph (ECG) revealed tachycardia.

8.1.1.3 Laboratory
- Blood leukocyte number was normal (WBC8.3 × 10^9/L).
- ESR (115 mm/h) and CRP (83.98 mg/L) were increased.
- IgG immunoglobulin (19.63 g/) was increased.
- Rheumatoid factor (4.7 IU/ml) was normal.

8.1.2 Imaging Examination

Chest X-ray (CXR) showed that there was a little cord shadow in the right lung, which could not explain the patient's condition. Considering that the patient is a young woman with high ESR and CRP, and clinically suspected vasculitis, in order to assess the vascular involvement of the patient, the cervical vessels of the patient were assessed by

J. Cao · Y. Wang · Z.-y. Jin (✉)
Department of Radiology, Peking Union Medical College Hospital, Chinese Academy of Medical Sciences and Peking Union Medical College, Beijing, China
e-mail: jinzy@pumch.cn

© Springer Nature Singapore Pte Ltd. 2020
Z.-y. Jin et al. (eds.), *Cardiac CT*, https://doi.org/10.1007/978-981-15-5305-9_8

color Doppler ultrasound, and the aortic and pulmonary arteries were assessed by CTA and CTPA.

8.1.2.1 X-Ray (Figs. 8.1, 8.2, and 8.3)

8.1.3 Imaging Findings and Diagnosis

The axial and postprocessing images of aorta and pulmonary CT angiography showed that both aorta and pulmonary artery were involved with multiple thickening of the wall and stenosis or occlusion of the lumen: left subclavian artery, left common carotid artery, brachiocephalic trunk, thoracic aorta, superior mesenteric artery, right upper and posterior pulmonary arteries, right middle lobe arteries and their branches. These changes are consistent with the manifestations of TAK diagnosis.

8.1.4 Management

- Medical therapy: systemic glucocorticoids plus glucocorticoid-sparing agent.
- Regular clinical follow-up (e.g., hematological examination, ultrasound, CT angiography).

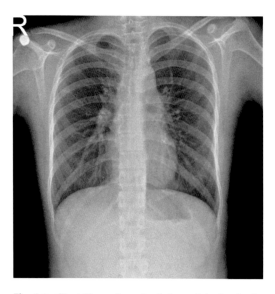

Fig. 8.1 Chest X-ray showed a little cord shadow in the right lung

8.2 Discussion

Takayasu's arteritis (TAK) is a kind of whole-layer arteritis with middle membrane damage and unknown cause [1].

The thickening and fibrosis of the whole wall of the artery were diffuse or irregular, which resulted in the stenosis and occlusion of the artery. In some cases, the aortic wall may swell to form spindle and/or saccular aneurysms due to the destruction of the middle membrane [2].

TAK is common in Asia and the Middle East. It occurs frequently in young women. About 80–90% of the patients are 20–30-years-old women [3]. The incidence and distribution of main affected arteries are different between men and women in different regions [4, 5]. In Japan and South America, carotid and thoracic aortas are more common, while in Israel and Asia, abdominal aorta and branches are more common. The most common symptoms of systemic inflammation are mild to moderate fever and asthenia, which are easy to be missed because of the unintentional clinical manifestations. The local symptoms were related to the location and degree of the involved vessels.

In patients with TAK, early detection and treatment of inflammatory or stenotic lesions can reduce associated morbidity and mortality [6]. For these patients, a biopsy is difficult or, many times, impossible. For this reason, the role of imaging in these patients is to aid in establishing the correct diagnosis, to determine the disease activity and extent, and also to monitor the treatment [7], correlation of imaging findings with the clinical data is mandatory.

8.3 Current Technical Status and Applications of CT

In patients with vasculitis, early detection and treatment of inflammatory or stenotic lesions can reduce associated morbidity and mortality. While conventional arteriography generally provides clear outlines of the lumen of involved arteries, it does not allow arterial wall thickening to be assessed and is an invasive test associated with some risks. Therefore, if a therapeutic interven-

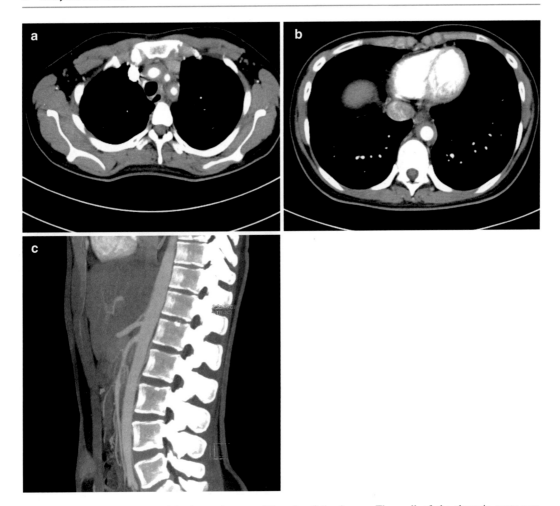

Fig. 8.2 Contrast-enhanced ECG-triggered aorta CT angiography performed on 2nd-generation dual-source CT. Contrast-enhanced axial images (**a–b**) showed left subclavian artery, left common carotid artery and brachiocephalic trunk with thickening of the wall and mild steno- sis of the lumen. The wall of the thoracic aorta was thickened and the lumen was mild stenosis. Maximum intensity projection image (**c**) showed local wall of the superior mesenteric artery was thickened and the lumen was moderate stenosis

tion (e.g., stenting for revascularization) is not anticipated, a less invasive imaging technique is preferred [8].

CTA can be used to assess the presence of luminal and perivascular changes. In active vasculitis, mural thickening with wall enhancement and a hypo-vascular halo have been described on delayed CT angiographic images. With inactive disease, mural calcifications with mild thickening and enhancement may be present. Stenosis, occlusion, and aneurysms may develop. One small study (25 patients) using CTA compared to conventional angiography for diagnosing TAK revealed a sensitivity and specificity of 100% [9]. Serial CT scans can be used to follow the response to treatment. The potential efficacy of this method was evaluated in 31 patients who underwent repeated CT angiography within 3 years [10]. At first, thoracic or abdominal aortic aneurysm was found in 12 patients (about 40%), and then 2 patients subsequently developed during follow-up. Despite glucocorticoid treatment, aneurysm size increased rapidly in three patients (more than 1 cm/year). This was accompanied by thickening of the wall, suggesting continued disease activity, leading to the rupture of the aorta.

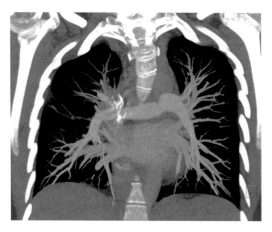

Fig. 8.3 Contrast-enhanced CT pulmonary angiography (CTPA) performed on 2nd-generation dual-source CT. Maximum intensity projection image showed the right upper and posterior pulmonary arteries, right middle lobe arteries and their branches were not seen

CT also allows the evaluation of pleural, pericardial, and lung involvement and aids in the detection of postoperative complications, such as paravalvular leakage or pseudoaneurysms.

CT angiography is superior in the evaluation of the coronary arteries and the peripheral branches of the pulmonary arteries and aorta. Cardiac CT provides an accurate assessment of the great vessels and coronary arteries, valve lesions, cardiac volumes, and cardiac function. Kang et al. reported that more than half of the patients with TAK in their study had coronary arterial lesions at coronary CTA, regardless of clinical symptoms and disease activity [11]. Coronary CTA performed with aortic CT angiography may yield additional information on coronary arterial lesions in patients with TAK.

The suggestions for technical and operational parameters on CT angiography in TAK is as follows [12]:

- Multislice CT scanner should be used.
- Collimation 0.6 mm, tube voltage 120 kV, tube current time product (mAs) determined by automatic dose modulation.

- Reconstruction slice thickness should be between 0.5 and 1.0 mm.
- Body-weight adapted injection of 60–120 mL of nonionic iodinated contrast agent ($\geq$350 mg/mL) using a power injector ($\geq$4 mL/s).
- Arterial phase: bolus-tracking method (threshold of 100 HU); ECG triggering.
- Venous phase: 50 s after finishing the arterial phase acquisition.

Compared with CTA, MRA has the advantage in that it does not use ionizing radiation and can be performed without the administration of intravenous contrast material. EULAR (European League Against Rheumatism) developed 12 recommendations on the use of imaging for the diagnosis and monitoring of large vessel vasculitis in 2018 [12]. It suggested that in patients with suspected TAK, MRI to investigate mural inflammation and/or luminal changes should be used as the first imaging test to make a diagnosis of TAK, and PET, CT, and/ or ultrasound may be used as alternative imaging modalities. A technique without radiation exposure is preferable over other modalities because of the young age of patients with TAK. Besides, MRI enables assessment of the vessel wall and luminal changes, which are both relevant for TAK. Ultrasound is of limited value for assessment of the thoracic aorta. This recommendation is almost entirely based on expert opinion and current clinical practice.

Hybrid imaging with FDG PET/MR imaging has also shown promise in these patients according to preliminary data, especially in large vessel vasculitis. The standard uptake values obtained with FDG PET/MR imaging correlated well with those obtained with FDG PET/CT. Also, the addition of the morphologic information of MR imaging to the FDG uptake values led to the detection of an increased number of affected segments, in comparison with PET or MR imaging alone [13, 14].

8.4   Key Points

- Takayasu's arteritis (TAK) is an uncommon chronic vasculitis of unknown etiology, which primarily affects the aorta and its primary branches.
- Early detection and treatment of inflammatory or stenotic lesions of TAK patients can reduce associated morbidity and mortality.
- Patients with suspected TAK should undergo imaging of the arterial tree of the chest, abdomen, head, and neck, or other areas demonstrates by CTA or MRA.

References

1. Isobe M. Takayasu arteritis revisited: current diagnosis and treatment. Int J Cardiol. 2013;168(1):3–10.
2. Rathod KR, Deshmukh HL, Garg AI, Mehta RC, Rachewad SS. Spectrum of angiographic findings in aortoarteritis. Clin Radiol. 2005;60(7):746–55.
3. Arend WP, Michel BA, Bloch DA, et al. The American College of Rheumatology 1990 criteria for the classification of Takayasu arteritis. Arthritis Rheum. 1990;33(8):1129.
4. Ishikawa K. Natural history and classification of occlusive thromboaortopathy (Takayasu's disease). Circulation. 1978;57(1):27.
5. Lupi-Herrera E, Sanchez-Torres G, Marcushamer J, Mispireta J, Horwitz S, Vela JE. Takayasu's arteritis. Clinical study of 107 cases. Am Heart J. 1977;93(1):94–103.
6. Broncano J, Vargas D, Bhalla S, et al. CT and MR imaging of cardiothoracic vasculitis. Radiographics. 2018;38:997–1021.
7. Pipitone N, Versari A, Salvarani C. Role of imaging studies in the diagnosis and follow-up of large-vessel vasculitis: an update. Rheumatology (Oxford). 2008;47(4):403–8.
8. Peter A Merkel. Clinical features and diagnosis of Takayasu arteritis – UpToDate 2019.
9. Yamada I, Nakagawa T, Himeno Y, et al. Takayasu arteritis: evaluation of the thoracic aorta with CT angiography. Radiology. 1998;209:103–9.
10. Sueyoshi E, Sakamoto I, Hayashi K. Aortic aneurysms in patients with Takayasu's arteritis: CT evaluation. AJR Am J Roentgenol. 2000;175:1727.
11. Kang E-J, Kim SM, Choe YH, et al. Takayasu arteritis: assessment of coronary arterialabnormalities with 128-section dual-source CT angiography of the coronary arteries and aorta. Radiology. 2014;270:74–81.
12. Dejaco C, Ramiro S, Duftne C, et al. EULAR recommendations for the use of imaging in large vessel vasculitis in clinical practice. Ann Rheum Dis. 2018;77(5):636–43.
13. Einspieler I, Thürmel K, Pyka T, et al. Imaging large vessel vasculitis with fully integrated PET/MRI: a pilot study. Eur J Nucl Med Mol Imaging. 2015;42(7):1012–24.
14. Grayson PC, Alehashemi S, Bagheri AA, et al. 18 F-Fluorodeoxyglucose-positron emission tomography as an imaging biomarker in a prospective, longitudinal cohort of patients with large vessel vasculitis. Arthritis Rheumatol. 2018;70(3):439. Epub 2018 Feb 6

Behcet's Disease

9

Jingwen Dai, Lu Lin, and Zheng-yu Jin

Abstract

Behcet's disease (BD) is a systemic vasculitis with a chronic, relapsing autoinflammatory condition that can involve both arteries and veins of any diameter and is characterized by manifestations affecting the skin, eyes, cardiovascular system, and gastrointestinal tract. Vascular involvement (vascular Behçet's disease; VBD) can lead to luminal stenosis, thrombus, and aneurysms and mainly affects the venous system usually with venous thrombosis as the initial presentation. Venous involvement in BD patients is far more common than arterial involvement. The typical form of arterial involvement is aneurysm. The abdominal aorta, the femoral artery, and the pulmonary artery are more commonly involved among arterial VBDs whereas coronary involvement is quite rare. In this chapter, based on a case of coronary pseudoaneurysm, we will discuss the imaging manifestations of VBDs involved with coronary artery.

J. Dai · L. Lin · Z.-y. Jin (✉)
Department of Radiology, Peking Union Medical College Hospital, Chinese Academy of Medical Sciences and Peking Union Medical College, Beijing, China
e-mail: jinzy@pumch.cn

9.1 Case of Behçet's Disease with Coronary Artery Pseudoaneurysms

9.1.1 History

- A 23-year-old male patient had intermittent chest pain irrelevant to exercise for the past 4 months and right lower abdominal pain with right lower limb swelling 10 days ago.
- He also had a history of recurrent oral aphthous for 10 years and a genital ulcer was newly found 1 week ago.

9.1.1.1 Physical Examination
- Blood pressure: 119/74 mmHg; Breathing rate: 18/min
- Heart rate: 85 bpm without arrhythmia

9.1.1.2 Echocardiogram and Ultrasonography
- Echocardiogram showed an enlargement of left atrium and hypokinesis of inferior and lateral wall of left ventricle.
- The results of lower limb ultrasonography indicated the thrombosis in the right external iliac vein and femoral vein.

9.1.1.3 Laboratory
- Erythrocyte sedimentation rate (ESR): 51 mm/h (elevated).
- NT-pro BNP: 582.8 pg/ml (elevated).

© Springer Nature Singapore Pte Ltd. 2020
Z.-y. Jin et al. (eds.), *Cardiac CT*, https://doi.org/10.1007/978-981-15-5305-9_9

- High sensitivity C reactive protein (hsCRP): 117.57 mg/L (elevated).
- Serum myocardial enzyme spectrum showed negative results.

9.1.2 Imaging Examination

9.1.2.1 CT Images

A coronary CT angiography was requested to investigate the coronary artery status (Fig. 9.1).

9.1.3 Imaging Findings and Diagnosis

The coronary CTA imaging results showed there was a huge pseudoaneurysm in the proximal and middle segment of RCA with thrombus inside. The distal segment of RCA was not well depicted. No significant stenosis has been found in LAD and LCX.

9.1.4 Management

- Medical therapy of prednisone, cyclophosphamide, and heparin
- Clinical follow-up of heart conditions

9.2 Discussion

Behcet's disease is a disorder characterized by chronic inflammation, with vasculitis as the pathological characteristic that results in multisystemic effects. Inflammatory responses involving arteries and veins are considered to be underlying pathology. Vascular involvement is a common complication in BD identified in about 40% of patients, accounting for the main cause of mortality. Arterial involvement is less common than venous involvement, as the arterial involvement accounts for 15%–20% of vascular complications [1]. Arterial involvement leads to a poor prognosis with death rates up to 13.5%, especially when the pulmonary artery and thoracic aorta are involved [2].

Cardiac involvement is one of the most lethal complications in BD with relatively high mortality. The manifestations of cardiac involvement in BD include pericarditis, coronary artery stenosis or aneurysm, myocardial infarction, myocarditis, endocarditis, and cardiomyopathy. Pericarditis is the most common type of cardiac involvement. It represents a wide spectrum of pericardial tamponade, constrictive pericarditis, acute pericarditis, or only pericardial effusion with no obvious symptoms [3, 4].

Coronary artery involvement is rare in Behcet's disease including coronary aneurysm, coronary stenosis, occlusion, and arteritis. Coronary aneurysms are more common with an incidence ranging from 1.5% to 5% [5]. Similar to the more severe manifestations of BD, the involvement of coronary artery is more frequent in male patients under 40 years old. Some of these coronary artery aneurysms are asymptomatic, while others can present as acute coronary syndrome, myocardial infarction, stable or unstable angina. The other diseases that can cause coronary aneurysm include Kawasaki disease, Takayasu arteritis, and atherosclerosis. Majority of the published cases about aneurysms manifestation of BD are discovered after BD was diagnosed, like in our case. Although in our case, the diagnosis of BD was undoubtable, atherosclerosis being an important risk factor for leading to aneurysm should always be taken into consideration, especially in old people with cardiac risk factors. But unlike other inflammatory systemic diseases, such as rheumatoid arthritis or systemic lupus erythematosus, BD does not accelerate the progression of atherosclerosis. Thus, in young patients presenting cardiac-related symptoms, but without obvious cardiovascular risk factors, cardiac involvement should be considered [6, 7].

Another manifestation of coronary artery involvement is coronary stenosis or occlusion results from fibrous intimal thickening caused by coronary arteritis [8]. This can lead to myocardial infarction, stable or unstable angina. In patients especially young patients without cardiovascular risk factors, nonatherosclerotic etiologies such as thrombosis arteritis and congenital abnormalities need to be considered. In BD, arteritis has been

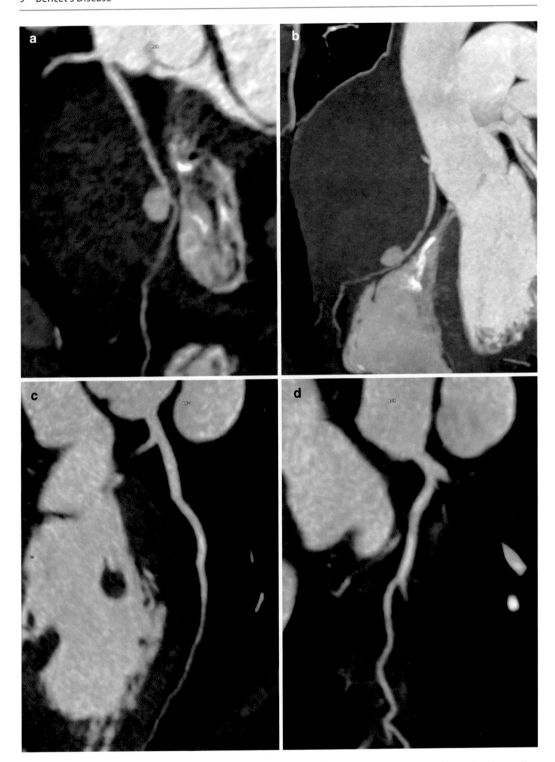

Fig. 9.1 Curved multi-planar (CPR) reconstructed images (**a**, right coronary artery [RCA]) and thin maximum intensity projection (MIP) image (**b**) of RCA shows a large pseudoaneurysm in the proximal and middle seg- ment of RCA. CPR image of left anterior descending [LAD] (**c**) and left circumflex artery [LCx] (**d**) shows no significant stenosis in both coronary arteries

considered as an independent pathophysiological factor for myocardial infarction.

It is important to assess whether there is cardiac involvement especially when the patients have cardiac-related clinical symptoms. BD patients with cardiac involvement have a poor prognosis compared to those without cardiac involvement [9].

In summary, although coronary artery aneurysm is a very uncommon manifestation in BD, it should be considered when young patients present chest pain. Since cardiac involvement leads to a poor prognosis, prompt diagnosis and systematic assessment are important.

9.3 Current Technical Status and Applications of CT

Multisystemic vasculitis is the main manifestation of Behcet's disease which can lead to thrombotic syndromes, aneurysmal arterial disease. CTA provides a structural assessment of arterial and venous vessels. It can evaluate the extent and severity of the cardiovascular involvement, delineating wall thickening, luminal stenosis, and aneurysmal dilation and also mural enhancement which was assumed to represent inflammatory activity. It can also demonstrate the abnormal of the target organ such as hemorrhage or infarction. CT may also be able to follow up on the development of vascular complications in BD patients.

For the BD patients who suspected to have coronary artery involvement, coronary CTA can noninvasively evaluate the abnormal anatomy and has showed an important role for these patients. However, the radiation dose of CTA limits its use especially in young patients and in follow-up imaging, but the development of low-dose CTA protocols may change this in the future.

9.4 Key Points

- Coronary artery involvement is rare in Behcet's disease including coronary aneurysm, coronary stenosis, occlusion, and arteritis.
- CTA plays an important role in evaluating the cardiac involvement and monitoring the development of the disease.

References

1. Duzgun N, Ates A, Aydintug OT, et al. Characteristics of vascular involvement in Behcet's disease. Scand J Rheumatol. 2006;35:65–8.
2. Saadoun D, Asli B, Wechsler B, et al. Long-term outcome of arterial lesions in Behcet disease: a series of 101 patients. Medicine. 2012;91:18–24.
3. Marzban M, Mandegar MH, Karimi A, et al. Cardiac and great vessel involvement in 'Behcet's disease. J Card Surg. 2008;23(6):765–8.
4. Kwon CM, Lee SH, Kim JH, et al. A case of Behcet's disease with pericarditis, thrombotic thrombocytopenic purpura, deep vein thrombosis and coronary artery pseudoaneurysm. Korean J Intern Med. 2006;21(1):50–6.
5. Pineda GE, Khanal S, Mandawat M, et al. Large atherosclerotic left main coronary aneurysm—a case report and review of the literature. Angiology. 2001;52(7):501–4.
6. Komooka M, Higashiue S, Matsubayashi K, et al. Vascular Behçet disease presenting large right coronary artery pseudoaneurysm after percutaneous coronary intervention (PCI): report of a case. Kyobu Geka. 2013;66:845–8.
7. Ugurlu S, Seyahi E, Yazici H. Prevalence of angina, myocardial infarction and intermittent claudication assessed by rose questionnaire among patients with Behcet's syndrome. Rheumatology. 2008;47:472–5.
8. Song MH, Watanabe T, Nakamura H. Successful off pump coronary artery bypass for Behcet's disease. Ann Thorac Surg. 2004;77(4):1451–4.
9. Geri G, Wechsler B, Huong DLT, et al. Spectrum of cardiac lesions in Behçet disease: a series of 52 patients and review of the literature. Medicine. 2012;91:25–34.

Kawasaki Disease

10

Rui Wang and Jianxing Qiu

Abstract

Kawasaki disease is an acute, self-limited systemic vasculitis, which occurs in infants and children predominantly. The etiology of Kawasaki disease is unknown. The diagnosis of Kawasaki disease is made based on the clinical findings. Kawasaki disease is characterized by fever, bilateral nonexudative conjunctivitis, mucocutaneous inflammation, changes in the rash, extremities, and cervical lymphadenopathy. The main complication is coronary artery aneurysms. If not treated early, one in five children develop coronary artery aneurysms, which may lead to ischemic heart disease or sudden death. Coronary artery aneurysms evolve dynamically over time. After illness onset, it usually reaches a peak dimension by 6 weeks. In the first 2 years, the risk of myocardial infarction caused by coronary artery thrombosis is highest. But stenosis and occlusion of coronary artery progress over years. The mortality in patients with giant aneurysms is very high. In young people, Kawasaki disease is no more a rare cause of acute coronary syndrome. If patients develop myocardial ischemia as a result of coronary artery aneurysms and stenosis, both percutaneous intervention and coronary artery bypass surgery can be used.

R. Wang · J. Qiu (✉)
Radiology Department, Peking University First Hospital, Beijing, China

10.1 Case of Kawasaki Disease

10.1.1 History

- A 10-year-old male patient presented to the hospital with a 1-week history of fever, rash, and arthralgia.

10.1.1.1 Physical Examination
- Blood pressure: 120/80 mmHg
- Breathing rate: 18/min
- Heart rate: 145 bpm
- Body temperature: 38.6 °C

10.1.1.2 Electrocardiograph
- Electrocardiography revealed sinus tachycardia (145 bpm)

10.1.1.3 Laboratory
- Anemia with a hemoglobin level: 89 g/l
- Elevated white blood cell count: 15.3×10^9/l
- Hypoalbuminemia: 30.4 g/l
- Elevated erythrocyte sedimentation rate: 25 mm/h
- Elevated C-reactive protein: 15 mg/l
- Urinalysis revealed sterile leukocyturia (20 cells/μl)
- Rheumatoid factor, antinuclear antibody, and serum angiotensin-converting enzyme levels: normal
- Blood and urine cultures and pharyngeal swab culture for *Streptococcus pyogenes*: negative.

Z.-y. Jin et al. (eds.), *Cardiac CT*, https://doi.org/10.1007/978-981-15-5305-9_10

- serological assays for hepatotropic viruses, human immunodeficiency virus, cytomegalovirus, Epstein–Barr virus: negative

10.1.2 Imaging Examination

10.1.2.1 CT Images

A coronary CT angiography (CCTA) was requested to investigate the coronary artery status.

10.1.3 Imaging Findings and Diagnosis

CT coronary angiography demonstrated aneurysms of LAD, LCX, and RCA (Fig. 10.1a). Figure 10.1b showed LAD aneurysm in the proximal segment about 2.4 cm long and about 9.0 mm in diameter, and calcified plaques in the aneurysm. (Fig. 10.1b). Dilatation of the proximal segment of the LCX was seen with a length of 0.9 cm and a maximum transverse diameter of about 6 mm (Fig. 10.1c). RCA showed an aneurysmal dilation in the proximal segment about 4.3 cm in length and 11 mm in diameter and calcified plaques in the aneurysm (Fig. 10.1d).

10.1.4 Management

- Usage of high-dose immunoglobulin infusion and oral aspirin
- Follow-up observations for coronary artery aneurysms

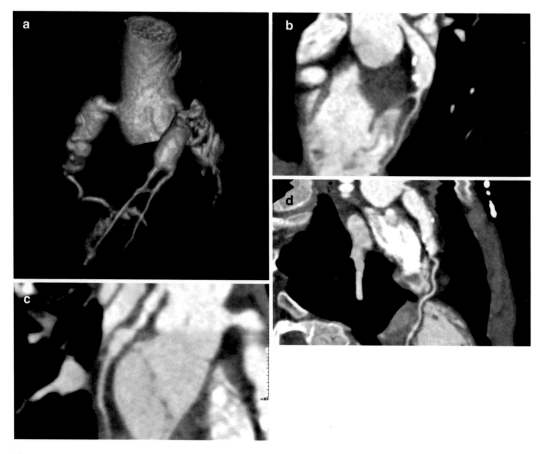

Fig. 10.1 Coronary tree (**a**) and curved multiplanar (CPR) reconstructed images (**b**, left anterior descending [LAD] branch; **c**, left circumflex artery [LCX]) and (**d**, right coronary artery [RCA]). (**a–d**) showed aneurysms of LAD, LCX, and RCA

10.2 Discussion

Kawasaki disease is an acute, self-limited systemic vasculitis, which occurs in infants and children predominantly. The diagnosis of Kawasaki disease is made based on the clinical findings. Manifested initially by fever, bilateral nonexudative conjunctivitis, mucocutaneous inflammation, changes in the rash, extremities, and cervical lymphadenopathy, Kawasaki disease aims at the coronary arteries and other cardiovascular structures [1].

The diagnosis of Kawasaki disease depends on the recognition of clinical criteria in the absence of a pathognomonic laboratory test [2]. Both meticulous history taking and thorough physical examination are the most significant factors in timely diagnosis and treatment. When the clinician suspects Kawasaki disease, clinical laboratory tests may be helpful in diagnosis and differential diagnosis.

The main complication is coronary artery aneurysms. The architecture of coronary artery aneurysms evolves dynamically over time [3]. After illness onset, it usually reaches a peak dimension by 6 weeks. In the first 2 years, the risk of myocardial infarction caused by coronary artery thrombosis is highest. But stenosis and occlusion of coronary artery progress over the years [4]. In the early months after illness onset, the natural history of aneurysms is closely related to the maximum extent of coronary enlargement and the number of coronary arteries involved [3, 5, 6].

The gold standard for diagnosis and follow-up of coronary artery aneurysms, thrombosis, and stenosis in patients with KD is selective invasive coronary angiography. Echocardiography, CT, and MRI are auxiliary diagnostic tools [7].

Kawasaki disease remains a poorly understood condition [8]. The diagnosis of Kawasaki disease depends mostly on clinical signs and symptoms. Proper treatment and follow-up are useful for its management. A rapid diagnosis and treatment can immensely help improve the prognosis and lower the associated complications of Kawasaki disease.

10.3 Current Technical Status and Applications of CT

For diagnosis and follow-up of coronary artery aneurysms, thrombosis, and stenosis in patients with Kawasaki disease, echocardiography is a noninvasive tool, but it does have some limitations, such as operator dependency, poor acoustic window, and poor ability to assess obstructive lesions and the distal portions of coronary arteries. Therefore, echocardiography is potential to lead to underestimation of disease severity. When echocardiography is suboptimal, no general consensus has been reached regarding the most acceptable diagnostic method for Kawasaki disease [9].

CT coronary angiography does not expose patients to the risk of possible procedural and vascular complications associated with invasive coronary angiography [10]. Moreover, CT can be performed without the need for hospitalization, which is required before and after invasive coronary angiography in order to administer intravenous anticoagulants. Compared with coronary MRI, ECG-gated multislice CT coronary angiography is an attractive alternative imaging technique for the younger patient. It can provide all required imaging results in terms of the number, size, and location of coronary aneurysms, necessary for diagnosis and follow-up [11].

The shape of coronary aneurysms may be elongated or spherical. And fusiform aneurysms may show "a string of beads" appearance or tortuosity. The diameter decreases gradually and reaches the normal diameter ultimately during aneurysm regression. Although after regression the appearance of coronary artery aneurysms becomes normal, the lumen may remain irregular. It can be a clue to the abnormal segments. CCTA can be used to evaluate obstructive lesions associated with coronary aneurysms, although the diagnostic accuracy still remains to be confirmed. Because of the beam hardening artifact and partial volume averaging effect, heavy calcification related to the aneurysm may make the accurate assessment of lumen patency by CCTA difficult. In coronary atherosclerotic disease, CT can be used to evaluate the patency of a bypass graft, which is placed to improve insufficient regional myocardial perfusion caused by obstructive coronary lesions of Kawasaki disease.

Conventional visualization techniques can be used, including multiplanar reformation, maximum intensity projection, and volume rendering. Better morphometric quantification of coronary arteries was provided by vessel analysis tools recently developed.

In summary, in patients with Kawasaki disease, CCTA is a useful tool to detect and monitor coronary artery abnormalities including artery aneurysm, stenosis, and occlusion. It also can reduce the frequency of more invasive diagnostic catheter coronary angiography.

10.4 Key Points

- Kawasaki disease is a pediatric vasculitis with coronary aneurysms as a major complication.
- Coronary CT angiography is a useful tool to detect and monitor coronary artery abnormalities including artery aneurysm, stenosis, and occlusion. It also can reduce the frequency of more invasive diagnostic catheter coronary angiography.

References

1. Kato H, Koike S, Yamamoto M, et al. Coronary aneurysms in infants and young children with acute febrile mucocutaneous lymph node syndrome. J Pediatr. 1975;86:892–8.
2. Newburger JW, Takahashi M, Gerber MA, et al. Diagnosis, treatment, and long-term management of Kawasaki disease: a statement for health professionals from the Committee on Rheumatic Fever, Endocarditis and Kawasaki Disease, Council on Cardiovascular Disease in the Young, American Heart Association. Circulation. 2004;110:2747–71.
3. Lin MT, Sun LC, Wu ET, et al. Acute and late coronary outcomes in 1073 patients with Kawasaki disease with and without intravenous γ-immunoglobulin therapy. Arch Dis Child. 2015;100:542–7.
4. Kato H, Sugimura T, Akagi T, et al. Long-term consequences of Kawasaki disease: a 10- to 21-year follow-up study of 594 patients. Circulation. 1996;94:1379–85.
5. Nakano H, Ueda K, Saito A, et al. Repeated quantitative angiograms in coronary arterial aneurysm in Kawasaki disease. Am J Cardiol. 1985;56:846–51.
6. Suzuki A, Kamiya T, Ono Y, et al. Follow-up study of coronary artery lesions due to Kawasaki disease by serial selective coronary arteriography in 200 patients. Heart Vessel. 1987;3:159–65.
7. Ghareep A, Alkuwari M, Willington F, et al. Kawasaki disease: diagnosis and follow-up by CT coronary angiography with the use of 128-slice dual source dual energy scanner. A case report. Pol J Radiol. 2015;80:526–8.
8. Jane W, Takahashi M, Jane C. Kawasaki Disease. J Am Coll Cardiol. 2016;67:1738–49.
9. Naiser JA, Schaller FA, Bannout R, et al. Kawasaki disease causing giant saccular aneurysm of the coronary arteries. Tex Heart Inst. 2008;35(3):369–70.
10. Aggarwala G, Iyengar N, Burke SJ. Kawasaki disease: role of coronary CT angiography. Int J Cardiovasc Imaging. 2006;22:803–5.
11. Goo HW, Park IS, Ko JK, et al. Coronary CT angiography and MR angiography of Kawasaki disease. Pediatr Radiol. 2006;36(7):697–705.

IgG4-Associated Coronary Artery Aneurysms

Qian Chen, Fan Zhou, and Longjiang Zhang

Abstract

IgG4-related disease is a unique immune-mediated fibroinflammatory condition, which is characterized by elevated serum IgG4 levels and tumefaction or tissue infiltration by IgG4-positive plasma cells. It can involve a wide variety of organs including the lung, kidney, liver, and exocrinological and endocrinological organs. The cardiovascular system is also a target of IgG4-related disease. Cases of IgG4-associated coronary artery involvement are rare. CCTA can accurately visualize the coronary artery involvement and monitor the therapeutic response. In this chapter, based on a case of IgG4-associated coronary artery aneurysm, we will discuss the cardiac CT imaging manifestations of the disease.

11.1 Case of IgG4-Associated Coronary Artery Aneurysms

11.1.1 History

- A 43-year-old male patient presented with acute chest pain for 2 days.

- He was admitted to the hospital and appointed to cardiac CT for suspected coronary artery disease (CAD).

11.1.1.1 Physical Examination
- Blood pressure: 140/100 mmHg; Breathing rate: 20/min
- Heart rate: 102 bpm without arrhythmia

11.1.1.2 Electrocardiograph
Standard 12-lead electrocardiograph (ECG) revealed ST-T segment elevation on leads II, III, AVF, V1–V5.

11.1.1.3 Laboratory Tests
- Serum myocardial enzyme spectrum showed negative results.
- Serum concentrations of IgG4 (5650 mg/dL) and C-reactive protein (78.1 mg/L) was abnormally high.

11.1.2 Imaging Examination

11.1.2.1 CT Images
A coronary CT angiography (CCTA) was requested to investigate the coronary artery status (Figs. 11.1 and 11.2).

Q. Chen · F. Zhou · L. Zhang (✉)
Department of Medical Imaging, Jinling Hospital,
Medical School of Nanjing University,
Nanjing, Jiangsu, China

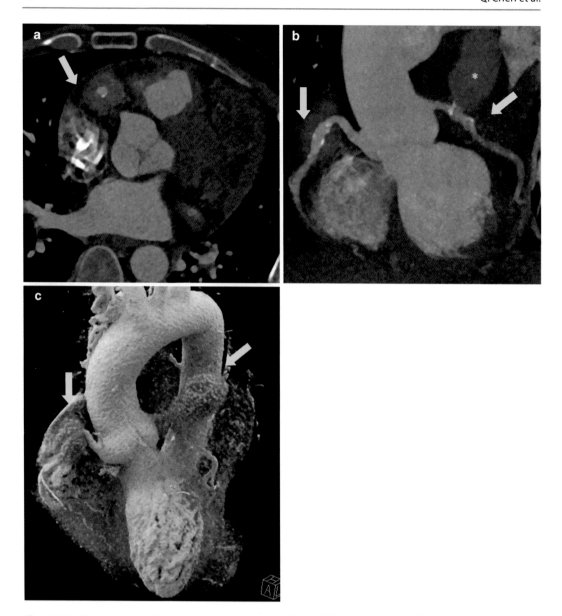

Fig. 11.1 Contrast-enhanced axial computed tomographic image (**a**) showing perivascular soft-tissue masses involving the right coronary artery (RCA) and left circumflex artery (LCX) (arrows). Maximum intensity projection reformatted image of CCTA (**b**) demonstrating perivascular soft-tissue masses involving the LCX and RCA (arrows) and a large aneurysm with a thrombus involving the left anterior descending (LAD) artery (asterisk). A three-dimensional rendering (**c**) demonstrated mass lesions involving the LAD and RCA (arrows)

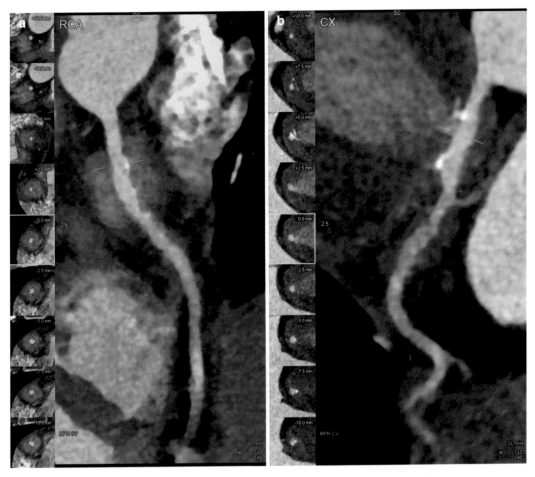

Fig. 11.2 Curved multi-planar (CPR) reconstructed images (**a, b**) show multiple soft-tissue masses in the epicardial space encasing the proximal segment of RCA and LCX. Mild-moderate luminal stenosis is seen in the proximal segment of LCX due to extrinsic compression by the mass

11.1.2.2 Conventional Coronary Angiography (Fig. 11.3)

11.1.3 Imaging Findings and Diagnosis

CCTA showed LCX and RCA were diffusely surrounded by tumor-like masses in the epicardial space. Mild-moderate luminal stenosis was seen in the proximal segment of LCX caused by extrinsic compression by the mass. CCTA demonstrated a huge aneurysmal lesion of LAD filled with massive intraluminal thrombi. PCI results showed a mass around the proximal segment of RCA and capillaries were seen in the mass. No obvious stenosis of RCA was found. Invasive coronary angiography demonstrated rupture of LM and contrast medium leakage from it. Fifty percent stenosis was detected in the proximal segment of LCX. LAD was not visualized on PCI images.

11.1.4 Management

- Coronary artery bypass graft surgery.
- Pathological examination of pericoronary mass (Fig. 11.4).

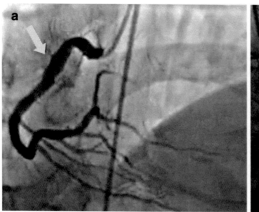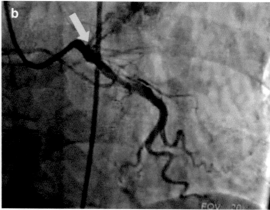

Fig. 11.3 Percutaneous transluminal coronary intervention (PCI) results. Invasive coronary angiography image for RCA (**a**) shows a mass surrounding the proximal segment of RCA and capillaries were seen in the mass (arrow). No obvious stenosis of RCA is found. Invasive coronary angiography image (**b**) demonstrates the rupture of LM and contrast medium leakage from it (arrow). 50% stenosis is detected in the proximal segment of LCX. LAD was not shown on PCI images

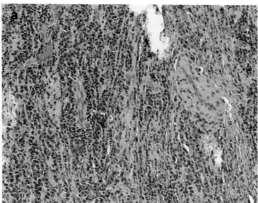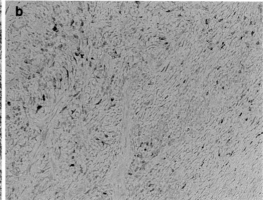

Fig. 11.4 Pathological examination showed infiltration of the coronary artery. Hematoxylin and Eosin staining (**a**) depicts widespread fibrosis and inflammatory change (×100). Immunohistochemical examination (**b**) reveals IgG4-expressing plasma cells in the coronary artery (×100)

11.2   Discussion

IgG4-related disease is a unique immune-mediated fibroinflammatory condition, which is characterized by elevated serum IgG4 levels and tumefaction or tissue infiltration by IgG4-positive plasma cells [1]. IgG4-related disease can affect various organs, such as pancreas, bile duct, lacrimal and salivary glands, thyroid, kidney, and lung [2]. The cardiovascular system is also a target of IgG4-related disease, which may be diagnosed incidentally or based on the cardiovascular symptoms [3].

Coronary artery engagement is described in only a limited number of cases so far. The infiltration of IgG4-positive plasmacytes occurs predominantly in the adventitial region, which can result in inflammatory pseudotumor, periarterial fibrosclerotic thickening, aneurysm, and artery stenosis [4]. They may lead to unfavorable outcomes such as myocardial infarction, dissection, aneurysmal rupture, and even death.

Diagnosis of IgG4-related disease is determined by histological findings that show IgG4-positive plasma cell and lymphocytic infiltration, storiform fibrosis, and obliterative phlebitis. High serum IgG4 level is an important hallmark for diagnosing IgG4-related disease [5]. The differential diagnosis should be systematic vasculitis involves coronary artery, such as Takayasu disease, Kawasaki disease, and Beçhet disease.

Myocardial infarction and/or arterial rupture can be fatal. Therefore, accurate evaluation of vascular involvement in IgG4-related disease using appropriate imaging modalities is important for optimal treatment planning (corticosteroid therapy vs. mechanical intervention vs. surgery) [6].

11.3 Current Technical Status and Applications of CT

Echocardiography should be used as a screening tool for the early detection of coronary artery involvement in IgG4-related disease patients [7]. FDG-PET is considered to be a useful tool for assessing organ involvement and monitoring the therapeutic response [8, 9]. Cardiac MR imaging can be performed to assess myocardial ischemia.

CCTA can accurately visualize the coronary involvement and monitor the therapeutic response [10]. Based on radiological findings observed in coronary arteries, vasculitic lesions are classified into three types as follows: stenotic, aneurysmal, and diffuse wall thickening [11]. The perivascular masses around the coronary arteries on CCTA resemble the shape of mistletoe. Mistletoe is a plant attached to the branches of a tree, similar to the perivascular soft tissue attached to the coronary tree. Therefore, a "mistletoe sign" is proposed for this disease on CCTA images [12]. The presence of the mistletoe sign at CCTA is probably rare, but it might be characteristic of retroperitoneal fibrosis. Therefore, the recognition of this sign could be of great importance, given the increasingly good long-term prognosis of this systemic disease.

11.4 Key Points

- IgG4-related disease can affect the cardiovascular system, including the coronary arteries.

- Multidetector CT is a useful noninvasive examination for establishing the primary diagnosis and defining the involvement of the coronary arteries, with typical findings of mistletoe sign.

References

1. Kamisawa T, Zen Y, Pillai S, et al. IgG4-related disease. Lancet. 2015;385(9976):1460–71.
2. Ozawa M, Fujinaga Y, Asano J, et al. Clinical features of IgG4-related periaortitis/periarteritis based on the analysis of 179 patients with IgG4-related disease: a case–control study. Arthritis Res Ther. 2017;19(1):223.
3. Mavrogeni S, Markousis-Mavrogenis G, Kolovou G. IgG4-related cardiovascular disease. The emerging role of cardiovascular imaging. Eur J Radiol. 86:169–75.
4. Satomi K, Yoh Z, Atsuhiro K, et al. Inflammatory abdominal aortic aneurysm: close relationship to IgG4-related periaortitis. Am J Surg Pathol. 2008;32(2):197.
5. Umehara H, Masaki Y, Kawano M, et al. Comprehensive diagnostic criteria for IgG4-related disease (IgG4-RD), 2011. Nippon Naika Gakkai Zasshi. 2012;22(1):21–30.
6. Tanigawa JM, Daimon MM, Murai MM, et al. Immunoglobulin G4–related coronary periarteritis in a patient presenting with myocardial ischemia. Hum Pathol. 2012;43(7):1131–4.
7. Komiya Y, Soejima M, Tezuka D, et al. Early detection and intervention of coronary artery involvement in immunoglobulin G4-related disease. Intern Med. 2017;57(4):617–22.
8. Nishimura S, Amano M, Izumi C, et al. Multiple coronary artery aneurysms and thoracic Aortitis associated with IgG4-related disease. Intern Med. 2016;55(12):1605.
9. Yabusaki S, Oyama-Manabe N, Manabe O, et al. Characteristics of immunoglobulin G4-related aortitis/periaortitis and periarteritis on fluorodeoxyglucose positron emission tomography/computed tomography co-registered with contrast-enhanced computed tomography. EJNMMI Res. 2017;7(1):20.
10. Xu X, Bai W, Ma H, et al. Remission of "mistletoe sign" after treatment. J Cardiovasc Comput Tomogr. 2019; https://doi.org/10.1016/j.jcct.2019.08.002.
11. Hourai R, Miyamura M, Tasaki R, et al. A case of IgG4-related lymphadenopathy, pericarditis, coronary artery periarteritis and luminal stenosis. Heart & Vessels. 2016;31(10):1–5.
12. Maurovichhorvat P. Coronary artery manifestation of Ormond disease: the "mistletoe sign". Radiology. 2017;282(2):160644.

Myocardial Bridging

12

Qian Chen, Fan Zhou, and Longjiang Zhang

Abstract

Myocardial bridging (MB) is a common congenital anomaly characterized by myocardial encasement of a coronary artery segment. It most commonly affects the mid-portion of the left anterior descending coronary artery (LAD). Coronary angiography (CAG) is commonly used for the diagnosis of MB, but with a low sensitivity. In recent years, coronary computed tomography angiography (CCTA) has been widely used in diagnosing MB. Typical findings associated with MB on CCTA include intramyocardial course of a coronary artery segment as well as the presence of the milking effect phenomenon. In this chapter, based on a case of MB, we will discuss the cardiac CT imaging manifestations of MB, and further possibly promising role of new cardiac CT technology in MB.

12.1 Case of MB

12.1.1 History

- A 52-year-old female patient had sudden chest pain for 2 days and chest tightness with syncope for 1 day.
- She was referred to perform a cardiac CT for suspected coronary artery disease (CAD).

Physical Examination
- Blood pressure: 123/78 mmHg; Breathing rate: 18/min
- Heart rate: 60 bpm without arrhythmia

Electrocardiograph
Standard 12-lead electrocardiograph (ECG) revealed a first-degree atrioventricular block.

Laboratory
- Serum myocardial enzyme spectrum showed negative results.

12.1.2 Imaging Examination

12.1.2.1 CT Images
CCTA and fractional flow reserve derived from CCTA (CT-FFR) were requested to investigate the coronary artery anatomical features and hemodynamic status (Figs. 12.1, 12.2, 12.3, and 12.4).

Q. Chen · F. Zhou · L. Zhang (✉)
Department of Medical Imaging, Jinling Hospital, Medical School of Nanjing University, Nanjing, Jiangsu, China

© Springer Nature Singapore Pte Ltd. 2020
Z.-y. Jin et al. (eds.), *Cardiac CT*, https://doi.org/10.1007/978-981-15-5305-9_12

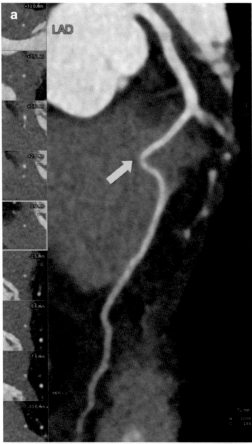

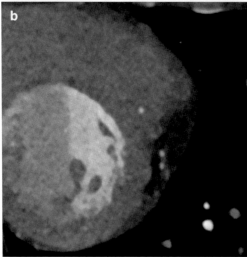

Fig. 12.1 Curved multi-planar (CPR) reconstructed image (**a**) and axial image (**b**) show deep myocardial bridging in the middle segment of LAD branch. The middle segment of LAD demonstrates mild stenosis. No plaque was seen in LAD

12.1.3 Imaging Findings and Diagnosis

The CCTA postprocessing images including CPR and VR results showed the middle segment of LAD was covered by myocardial tissue. The middle segment of LAD demonstrated mild stenosis. No plaque can be seen in LAD. CT-FFR image demonstrated decreased FFR value in the segment distal to MB which indicated impaired hemodynamic status.

12.1.4 Management

- Out-patient follow-up observations for MB.

12.2 Discussion

MB is a segment of the myocardium covering a coronary artery, while the tunneled artery is termed a mural coronary artery (MCA) [1]. MB is the commonest congenital coronary abnormality, with a prevalence of 0.5–11.8% on coronary angiography and 4–58% on CT [2], and is associated with hypertrophic cardiomyopathy with a prevalence as high as 30% [3].

MB is most frequently localized to the middle segment of the LAD artery on coronary angiography; however, other major coronary arteries can also be involved. Typical MB depth is reported at 1–10 mm, with a length of 10–30 mm [4]. MB of the LAD artery found on pathology has been characterized by Ferreira as falling into two distinct subtypes: superficial muscle type and deep muscle type [5]. The former does not constrict the coronary flow during systole; whereas the latter may compress the coronary artery, reduce the flow, and induce myocardial ischemia.

MB does not produce any symptoms in most patients. However, conditions which increase the amount of systolic compression (e.g., hypertrophic cardiomyopathy) and/or decrease diastolic filling disproportionately (e.g., rapid

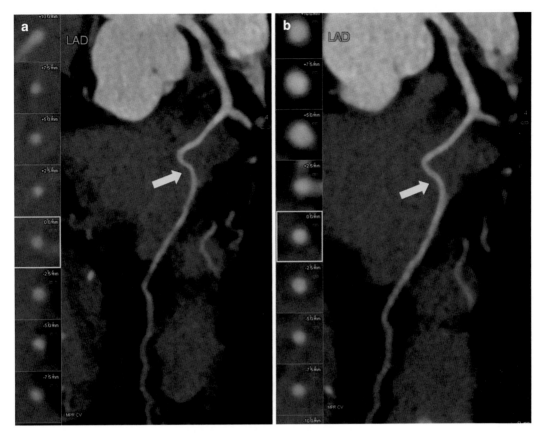

Fig. 12.2 The mural coronary of LAD in different cardiac cycles. CPR images of LAD show mild stenosis in the systolic phase (**a**) and no stenosis in the diastolic phase (**b**)

heart rates) may exacerbate the myocardial oxygen supply/demand mismatch, resulting in ischemic complications such as acute coronary syndromes, arrhythmias, coronary vasospasm, left ventricular dysfunction, and even sudden death [6].

Patients may require treatment when their symptoms may be attributable to MB. In drug-refractory cases, before the patient proceeds to percutaneous or surgical intervention, the presence of objective ischemia in the corresponding myocardial territory should be documented by diagnostic modalities such as isotope stress testing [7]. It is, therefore, important to evaluate its hemodynamics to determine management strategy, particularly in symptomatic patients without concomitant CAD.

12.3 Current Technical Status and Applications of CT

During the past decade, technological advances such as CCTA and intravascular ultrasound have contributed greatly to our understanding of the anatomic, hemodynamic, and pathophysiological consequences of MB.

The currently available multi-detector CT scanners with a high temporal resolution allow visualization of the vessel lumen during most of the cardiac cycle, making dynamic CT imaging of MB possible [8]. It can accurately determine the location, depth, and length of MB and visualize the characteristic milking effect of MB [9]. However, CCTA is unable to accurately assess the hemodynamic relevance of MB.

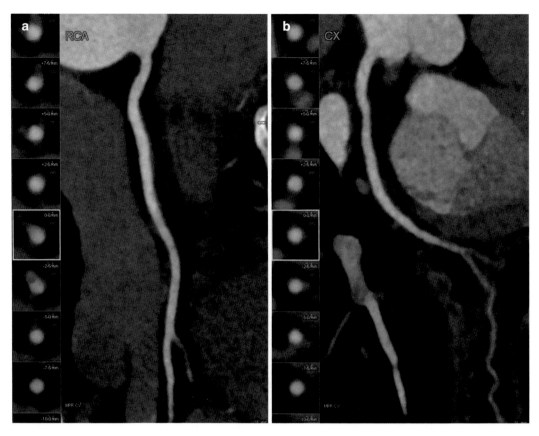

Fig. 12.3 Curved multi-planar (CPR) reconstructed images (**a, b**) show no stenosis in the right coronary artery (RCA) and left circumflex artery (LCX)

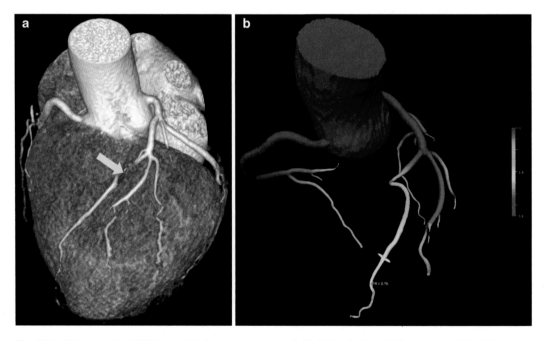

Fig. 12.4 Volume render (VR) image (**a**) shows deep myocardial bridging in the middle segment of the left anterior descending (LAD) branch. CT-FFR image (**b**) demonstrates decreased FFR value (0.72) in the segment distal to MB

Transluminal attenuation gradient (TAG) is defined as the transluminal opacification gradient of proximal to distal vessels in computed tomography. TAG shows a linear correlation with the extent of intracoronary transluminal stenosis [10]. It has been identified that an optimal cutoff value of TAG as −18.8 HU/10 mm is a better predictor of MB with systolic compression ≥50%, compared to the length or depth of the MB [11].

Recently, perfusion imaging approach has become more and more prevail in the clinical application. Coronary CTA combined with stress myocardial CT perfusion enable to assess the morphologic abnormalities and hemodynamic significance simultaneously [12]. It may help guide therapeutic strategies and posttreatment assessments in the future [13].

CT-FFR has been used for the noninvasive assessment of lesion-specific ischemia and has shown high diagnostic performance in patients with stable CAD. It offers a noninvasive method for evaluating the hemodynamic status in MB patients with high diagnostic performance [14, 15]. CT-FFR has shown promise in predicting proximal plaque formation in MB patients, which may guild early intervention in the future [16].

12.4   Key Points

- MB may present with chest pain similar to those with CAD or in acute coronary syndromes.
- Appropriate cardiac CT examination with developing advanced imaging technologies may contribute to the diagnosis of MB and evaluation of hemodynamic status.

References

1. Angelini P, Velasco JA, Flamm S. Coronary anomalies: incidence, pathophysiology, and clinical relevance. Circulation. 2002;105(20):2449–54.

2. Hazirolan T, Canyigit M, Karcaaltincaba M, et al. Myocardial bridging on MDCT. AJR Am J Roentgenol. 2007;188(4):1074–80.

3. Lee MS, Chen CH. Myocardial bridging: an up-to-date review. J Invasive Cardiol. 2015;27(11):521–8.

4. Angelini P, Trivellato M, Donis J, et al. Myocardial bridges: a review. Prog Cardiovasc Dis. 1983;26(1):75–88.

5. Ferreira AJ, Trotter SE, Konig BJ, et al. Myocardial bridges: morphological and functional aspects. Br Heart J. 1991;66(5):364–7.

6. Alegria JR, Herrmann J, Holmes DR Jr, et al. Myocardial bridging. Eur Heart J. 2005;26(12):1159–68.

7. Bruschke AVG, Veltman CE, Graaf MAD, et al. Myocardial bridging: what have we learned in the past and will new diagnostic modalities provide new insights? Neth Heart J. 2013;21(1):6–13.

8. Flohr TG, Mccollough CH, Bruder H, et al. First performance evaluation of a dual-source CT (DSCT) system. Eur Radiol. 2006;16(2):256–68.

9. Zhang LJ, Yang GF, Zhou CS, et al. Multiphase evaluation of myocardial bridging with dual-source computed tomography. Acta Radiol. 2009;50(7):775–80.

10. Choi JH, Min JK, Labounty TM, et al. Intracoronary transluminal attenuation gradient in coronary CT angiography for determining coronary artery stenosis. J Am Coll Cardiol Img. 2011;4(11):1149–57.

11. Yu M, Zhang Y, Li Y, et al. Assessment of myocardial bridge by cardiac CT: intracoronary transluminal attenuation gradient derived from diastolic phase predicts systolic compression. Korean J Radiol. 2017;18(4):655–63.

12. Danad I, Szymonifka J, Schulman-Marcus J, et al. Static and dynamic assessment of myocardial perfusion by computed tomography. Eur Heart J Cardiovasc Imaging. 2016;17(8):836–44.

13. Lim JW, Lee H, Her K, et al. Myocardial CT perfusion imaging for pre- and postoperative evaluation of myocardial ischemia in a patient with myocardial bridging: a case report. Medicine. 2017;96(42):e8277.

14. Zhou F, Tang CX, Schoepf UJ, et al. Fractional flow reserve derived from CCTA may have a prognostic role in myocardial bridging. Eur Radiol. 2019;29(6):3017–26.

15. Zhou F, Wang YN, Schoepf UJ, et al. Diagnostic performance of machine learning based CT-FFR in detecting ischemia in myocardial bridging and concomitant proximal atherosclerotic disease. Can J Cardiol. 2019;35(11):1523–33.

16. Zhou F, Zhou CS, Tang CX, et al. Machine learning using CT-FFR predicts proximal atherosclerotic plaque formation associated with LAD myocardial bridging. JACC Cardiovasc Imaging. 2019;12(8):1591–3.

Coronary Artery Origin Anomalies (CAOA)

Kai Zhao and Jianxing Qiu

Abstract

Congenital coronary artery abnormalities are uncommon but can lead to chest pain or even sudden cardiac death in some cases of hemodynamic abnormalities. Among all the congenital abnormalities, coronary artery origin anomalies (CAOA) is considered to be one with the highest risk of sudden cardiac death (SCD) in young athletes. CAOA include either the right coronary artery originating from the left aortic sinus, which is reported to be more common; or the left coronary arising from the right sinus of Valsalva. Advanced imaging is an important and essential tool to define anatomic characteristics of anomalous aortic origin of coronary arteries. For decades, conventional cardiac angiography has been used to diagnose CAOA. The development of ECG-gated multi-detector row computed tomography (CT) has made it possible to describe the origin and proximal path of abnormal coronary arteries accurately and noninvasively.

13.1 Case of CAOA

13.1.1 History

- A 16-year-old young female patient had discontinuous dizziness in the past 6 years.
- She became unconscious twice in the past 6 years.
- She appointed to cardiac CTA.

Physical Examination
- Blood pressure: 108/67 mmHg
- Postural orthostatic tachycardia

Electrocardiograph
- Standard 12-lead electrocardiograph (ECG) revealed sinus rhythm with Left axis deviation.

Laboratory
- All the laboratory tests showed negative results.

13.1.2 Imaging Examination

CT and MR Images
A coronary CT angiography (CTA) and a cardiac MR was requested to investigate the coronary artery and myocardium (Figs. 13.1 and 13.2).

K. Zhao · J. Qiu (✉)
Radiology Department, Peking University First
Hospital, Beijing, China

© Springer Nature Singapore Pte Ltd. 2020
Z.-y. Jin et al. (eds.), *Cardiac CT*, https://doi.org/10.1007/978-981-15-5305-9_13

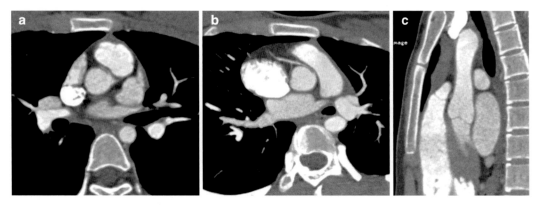

Fig. 13.1 Multi-planar (MPR) reconstructed images to show the right coronary artery (RCA) arising from the left sinus of Valsalva on computed tomography coronary angiography. Severe proximal stenosis of RCA could be seen. (**a, b, c**) Coronary CTA images

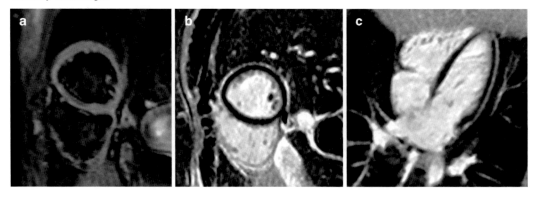

Fig. 13.2 Cardiac MR images. (**a**) Black blood sequence with fat suppression, short axis view; (**b**) Late Gadolinium Enhanced (LGE) sequence, short axis view; (**c**) LGE sequence, Four-chamber view. No significant abnormal signal has been shown in the images

13.1.3 Imaging Findings and Diagnosis

The coronary CTA images results showed RCA originate from the left coronary sinus and take an interarterial course between the pulmonary artery and the aorta. The Vascular lumen during the interarterial course is severe stenosis. When the aorta dilates during exercise, the abnormal slit-like ostium of RCA in the left sinus becomes narrower, restricting coronary blood flow and leading to myocardial infarction possibly. Fortunately, for this young patient, four-chamber views, two-long chamber views, and two-short chamber views of the cardiac MR images, no significant myocardial edema, myocarditis, and myocardial infarction was shown. A variation type is that the right coronary arises from the superior border of the left sinus of Valsalva or from above left sinus of Valsalva (Fig. 13.3).

13.1.4 Management

- Consultation of cardiac surgery department, and surgical interference should be taken if necessary.
- Avoid strenuous exercise; avoid long-time standing.

13.2 Discussion

The coronary artery anomalies are classified into anomalies of origin, anomalies of course, and anomalies of termination. and its pathophysiol-

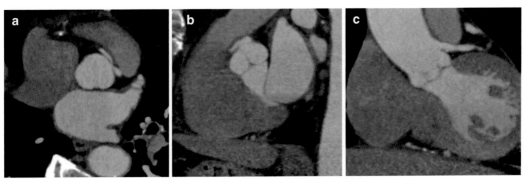

Fig. 13.3 Multi-planar (MPR) reconstructed images of another patient with anomalous aortic origin of the right coronary artery arising from above the left sinus of Valsalva on computed tomography coronary angiography. (**a**, **b**, **c**) Coronary CTA images

ogy, clinical manifestation, and significance are different.

CAOA is the second leading cause of SCD among young athletes and is responsible for 15%–20% of sudden deaths in this population [1, 2]. The risk of SCD is the highest in young people, especially during or after strenuous exercise. The true prevalence of CAOA in the general population remains unknown, and most research focused on patients with symptoms. Studies that focused on adult cohorts showed a very low mortality rate (<1%) after 1–5 years of follow-up [3].

The typical symptoms for patients with CAOA are exertional chest pain, palpitations, syncope, and even SCD [3]. Multiple pathophysiological mechanisms have been proposed for the occurrence of SCD [4], which include occlusion and/or compression of the abnormal coronary with intramural segment or interarterial course, especially during or after exercise, leading to myocardial ischemia or ventricular arrhythmias.

Advanced imaging methods, including computed tomography angiography and cardiac magnetic resonance imaging, are very helpful in figuring out the anatomy of CAOA, including ostial morphology, interarterial, intramural, or intramyocardial course. Cardiac catheterization combined with intravascular ultrasound was used to evaluate the degree of coronary stenosis [3, 4].

The lack of prospective and long-term data makes it tough to manage these patients with CAOA. The current statement and guideline [5, 6] recommend to distinguish high-risk CAOA from the recognized low-risk one. Intervention is not recommended for asymptomatic patients. And surgical intervention is provided for high-risk symptomatic patients.

13.3   Current Technical Status and Applications of CT

The diagnosis and treatment of coronary artery abnormality are various. A multidisciplinary team including cardiologists, cardiovascular surgeons, cardiovascular radiologists, nurses, and researchers should be developed [3].

Cross-sectional imaging such as CT or MRI plays an important role in the detection, classification, and risk stratification of patients with CAOA. Some patients are diagnosed by transthoracic echocardiography (TTE), but more and more patients are confirmed by CTA. Meanwhile, anatomical details and the diagnosis is usually made or confirmed by cross-sectional imaging.

CTA is a reliable method to image coronary arteries. Due to the overlapping helical techniques and iterative reconstructions [7], the new generation of CT scanners reduced the dose of ionic radiation by 60%–90% compared to the older ones. The cumulative dose of CTA is about 2–5 mSv, which is lower than the dose of coronary catheterization. It has been reported that CTA may be superior to conventional cardiac angiography in determining and showing the origin and proximal path of abnormal branches of coronary arteries [8]. Understanding the CT signs of coronary artery anomalies and their clinical significance is very important for accurate diagnosis and treatment of patients.

Myocardial perfusion assessment has become an important part of assessing risk stratification patients with CAOA. Some hospitals use stress echocardiography or stress CTA to identify wall motion anomalies. The advantage of MRI is that it provides information about myocardial function, perfusion, viability, and blood flow without ionizing radiation. It can provide high-quality cardiac imaging with good spatial resolution, and has better sensitivity and specificity [9].

13.4 Key Points

- CAOA is considered to be with a high risk of SCD in young athletes.
- Understanding the CT manifestations of various coronary artery anomalies and the clinical significance of these anomalies is critical for accurate diagnosis and appropriate patient treatment.

References

1. Basso C, Maron BJ, Corrado D, et al. Clinical profile of congenital coronary artery anomalies with origin from the wrong aortic sinus leading to sudden death in young competitive athletes. J Am Coll Cardiol. 2000;35:1493–501.
2. Maron Barry J, Doerer Joseph J, Haas Tammy S, et al. Sudden deaths in young competitive athletes. Circulation. 2009;119:1085–92.
3. Molossi S, Sachdeva S. Anomalous coronary arteries: what is known and what still remains to be learned? Curr Opin Cardiol. 2020;35(1):42–51.
4. Poynter JA, Williams WG, McIntyre S, et al. Anomalous aortic origin of a coronary artery: a report from the congenital heart surgeons society registry. World J Pediatr Congenit Heart Surg. 2014;5(1):22–30.
5. Van Hare GF, Ackerman MJ, Evangelista JA, et al. Eligibility and disqualification recommendations for competitive athletes with cardiovascular abnormalities: task force 4: congenital heart disease: a scientific statement from the American Heart Association and American College of Cardiology. Circulation. 2015;132:e281–91.
6. Brothers JA, Frommelt MA, Jaquiss RD, et al. Expert consensus guidelines: anomalous aortic origin of a coronary artery. J Thorac Cardiovasc Surg. 2017;153:1440–57.
7. Kim SY, Seo JB, Do KH, et al. Coronary artery anomalies: classification and ECG-gated multi-detector row CT findings with angiographic correlation. Radiographics. 2006;26(2):317–33.
8. Shi H, Aschoff AJ, Brambs HJ, et al. Multislice CT imaging of anomalous coronary arteries. Eur Radio. 2004;14:2172–81.
9. Agrawal H, Mery C, Krishnamurthy R, et al. Stress myocardial perfusion imaging in anomalous aortic origin of a coronary artery: results following a standardized approach. J Am Coll Cardiol. 2017;69(11_S):1616.

Coronary Artery Fistula

14

Kang Zhou, Yining Wang, and Zheng-yu Jin

Abstract

Coronary artery fistulas (CAF) are abnormal terminations of the coronary arteries. CAFs are direct connections between a coronary artery and a cardiac chamber or a vessel close to the heart. The clinical characteristic of CAFs is dependent on the severity of the left-to-right shunt. Most adult patients are usually asymptomatic. If a large left-to-right shunt exists, congestive heart failure, pulmonary hypertension, and rupture or thrombosis of the fistula may occur in early life. Correct and early diagnosis of coronary artery fistulas is important, and early surgical correction is indicated because of the high prevalence of late symptoms and complications. Traditionally, conventional angiography was the gold standard for the diagnosis of coronary anomalies. With more frequent use of multidetector computed tomography (CT) in chest and cardiac imaging, the incidence of coronary artery fistulas has been increasing.

14.1 Case of CAF

14.1.1 History

A 23-year-old male patient felt progressive exertional chest tightness for the past 4 years, edema of lower limbs for 1 year.

Physical Examination
- Body temperature: 36.2 °C; SpO2 98%; Blood pressure: 100/65 mmHg; Breathing rate: 18/min; Heart rate: 102 bpm without arrhythmia
- 4/6 double-phase murmur in the fourth intercostal space of the left sternal margin
- Anemia appearance

Electrocardiograph
Small Q-waves in II, III, and avF leads.

Laboratory
Serum myocardial enzyme spectrum showed negative results.

14.1.2 Imaging Examination

CT images
A coronary CT angiography (CTA) was requested to investigate the coronary artery status (Fig. 14.1).

K. Zhou · Y. Wang · Z.-y. Jin (✉)
Department of Radiology, Peking Union Medical
College Hospital, Chinese Academy of Medical
Sciences and Peking Union Medical College,
Beijing, China
e-mail: jinzy@pumch.cn

© Springer Nature Singapore Pte Ltd. 2020
Z.-y. Jin et al. (eds.), *Cardiac CT*, https://doi.org/10.1007/978-981-15-5305-9_14

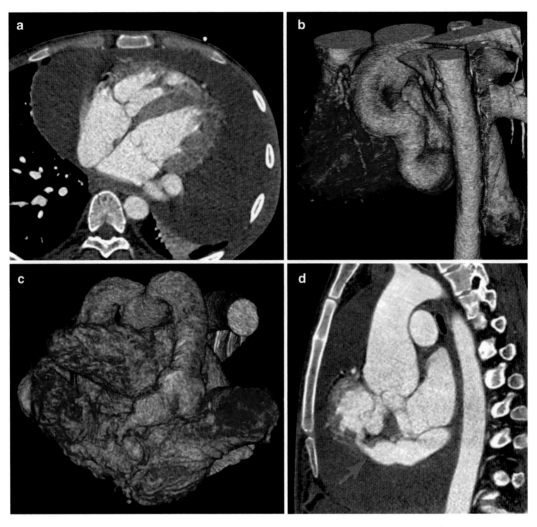

Fig 14.1 (**a**) Axial image showed a large amount of pericardial effusion. (**b**, **c**) volume rendering (VR) images showed a large fistula vessel originated from the left circumflex artery (LCX) and drainaged to the right ventricle. (**d**) maximum intensity projection image could verify the drainage site of CAF (arrow)

Conventional Coronary Angiography (Fig. 14.2)

14.1.3 Management

- This patient received surgery after diagnosis; the coronary artery fistula vessel has been closed, and a bypass between the left internal mammary artery and left anterior descending artery was built.

14.1.4 Imaging Findings and Diagnosis

The coronary CTA images results showed LCA-RV fistula with a large fistula vessel. Coexistent abnormalities were both ventricular enlargements and pericardial effusion. The large amount of pericardial effusion was revealed clearly on the axial images. Both ventricular enlargements can be identified on axial, MIP, and

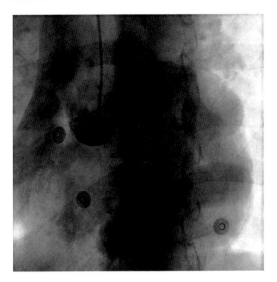

Fig 14.2 Conventional angiography was performed with a pigtail catheter at the root of the aorta. A very large abnormal vessel was observed; it originated from the root of the aorta and went along the margin of the heart. The drainage site was within the reign of the heart, but the exact location was not clear.

VR images. The route of the fistula vessel can be observed on the VR images conveniently. The origin site and drainage site of the fistula can be observed and measured on the MIP images accurately.

14.2 Discussion

CAFs are direct connections between a coronary artery and a cardiac chamber or a vessel close to the heart [1]. CAF was first described in 1865 by Krause [2]. CAF can be congenital or acquired; most CAFs are congenital form. CAFs are 0.002% in the general population but present in 0.05%–0.25% of patients who received coronary angiography [3–5]. The clinical presentation of CAFs is mainly dependent on the severity of the left-to-right shunt. The majority of adult patients are usually symptomatic. If a large left-to-right shunt exists, complications could be orthopnea, fatigue, endocarditis, chest pain, stroke, arrhythmias, myocardial ischemia, pulmonary hyperten-

sion, myocardial infarction, congestive heart failure, and rupture or thrombosis of the fistula or associated arterial aneurysm, and rarely, these presenting features can lead to sudden death [4, 6–8]. Early diagnosis and surgical correction are important for patients with large left-to-right shunt. Coronary angiography can precisely demonstrate the proximal part of the CAF and evaluate the size and number of fistulas, but because of significant dilution of the contrast medium, the drainage sites may not be well-visualized [9]. Only markedly enlarged coronary fistula vessel can be detected with echocardiography [10]. CT is a noninvasive and accurate imaging method for the detection of CAFs. Multidetector CT can provide high-resolution anatomic images of the whole heart. Use of multiplanar reformation can demonstrate sites of origin and drainage of fistula vessel. Volume rendering images provide an excellent overview of the cardiac and vascular anatomy which can help surgeons to do the plan before surgery [11].

14.3 Current Technical Status and Applications of CT

Recently, coronary multidetector CT has become a widely used technique that has proven useful to evaluate the cardiovascular anatomy and anomalies. The routine protocol of coronary CTA with electrocardiographically gated reconstruction methods can hold the demand for diagnosis. Sometimes, the fistula drainage to a rare site, such as superior vena cava, bronchial Arteries, a larger field of view (FOV) is needed for the scan protocol.

14.4 Key Points

- CAF is a rare kind of coronary abnormality. Most adult patients with CAF are usually asymptomatic. The CAF patients with severe left-to-right shunt have life-threatening complications, early diagnosis and surgical management is important.

- Multidetector CTA can provide high-resolution anatomic images for diagnosis and demonstrating sites of origin and drainage of fistula vessel.

References

1. Schumacher G, Roithmaier A, Lorenz HP, et al. Congenital coronary artery fistula in infancy and childhood: diagnostic and therapeutic aspects. Thorac Cardiovasc Surg. 1997;45(6):287–94.
2. Krause W. Uber den ursprung einer accessorischena. coronaria aus der a. pulmonalis. Z Ratl Med. 1865;24:225–7.
3. Chen CC, Hwang B, Hsiung MC, et al. Recognition of coronary arterial fistula by Doppler 2-dimensional echocardiography. Am J Cardiol. 1984;53(2):392–4.
4. Balanescu S, Sangiorgi G, Castelvecchio S, et al. Coronary artery fistulas: clinical consequences and methods of closure. Ital Heart J. 2001;2(9):669–76.
5. Kamineni R, Butman SM, Rockow JP, et al. An unusual case of an accessory coronary artery to pulmonary artery fistula: successful closure with transcatheter coil embolization. J Interv Cardiol. 2004;17(1):59–63.
6. Said SA, Lam J, van der Werf T. Solitary coronary artery fistulas: a congenital anomaly in children and adults. Congenit Heart Dis. 2006;1(3):63–76.
7. Wang NK, Hsieh LY, Shen CT, Lin YM. Coronary arteriovenous fistula in pediatric patients: a 17-year institutional experience. J Formos Med Assoc. 2002;101(3):177–82.
8. Rittenhouse EA, Doty DB, Ehrenhaft JL. Congenital coronary artery-chamber fistula: review of operative management. Ann Thorac Surg. 1975;20(4):468–85.
9. Schmitt R, Froehner S, Brunn J, et al. Congenital anomalies of the coronary arteries: imaging with contrast-enhanced, multi-detector computed tomography. Eur Radiol. 2005;15(6):1110–21.
10. Gowda RM, Vasavada BC, Khan IA. Coronary artery fistulas: clinical and therapeutic considerations. Int J Cardiol. 2006;107(1):7–10.
11. Taoka Y, Nomura M, Harada M, et al. Coronarypulmonary artery fistulas depicted by multiplanar reconstruction using magnetic resonance imaging. Jpn Circ J. 1998;62(6):455–7.

Anomalous Pulmonary Venous Connections

15

Yang Gao and Bin Lu

Abstract

Anomalous pulmonary venous connections (APVC) refers to single or multiple pulmonary veins that are not drawn into the anatomic left atrium, but directly into the systemic venous and right atrial. Partial or all pulmonary veins abnormally connected with the right atrial or systemic vein will result in volume overload of the right heart. The physiological effect is left-to-right shunt which is quite similar to that of an atrial septal defect (ASD). In most cases, the presence of ASD is accompanied by an anomalous pulmonary venous connection. The type of partial anomalous pulmonary venous connection is more common. According to the location of the abnormal connection of pulmonary vein, it is divided into the super-cardiac type, the intra-cardiac type, and the sub-cardiac type. The right upper pulmonary vein connecting to the superior vena cava is the most common, which belongs to the super-cardiac type. The intra-cardiac type refers to the pulmonary veins abnormally drawn into the right atrial or the coronary sinus ostium. The sub-cardiac type defined as the pulmonary veins abnormally drawn into the inferior vena cava or hepatic vein. Cardiac imaging with CTA or CMR is ideal for delineating pulmonary venous connections. Echocardiography is an important part of the evaluation of intracardiac malformation, and may identify the anomalous veins particularly in patients with excellent acoustic windows; however, CTA is superior for evaluating extracardiac vascular anatomy with excellent spatial resolution and volume rendering reconstruction.

15.1 Case of APVC

15.1.1 History

- A 19-year-old female patient discovered a heart murmur for more than a month.
- There was no obvious cyanosis or hypoxia after activity.

Physical Examination
- Blood pressure: 94/60 mmHg; Breathing rate: 20/min; Heart rate: 83 bpm
- 3/6 grade systolic wind—like murmurs are audible in the intercostal 2–3 on the left margin of the sternum.

15.1.2 Imaging Examination

Chest Radiography

Y. Gao · B. Lu (✉)
Department of Radiology, Fuwai Hospital, Chinese Academy of Medical Sciences and Peking Union Medical College, Beijing, China

© Springer Nature Singapore Pte Ltd. 2020
Z.-y. Jin et al. (eds.), *Cardiac CT*, https://doi.org/10.1007/978-981-15-5305-9_15

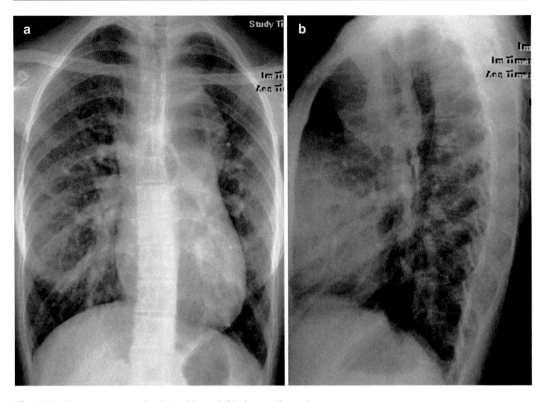

Fig. 15.1 X-ray anteroposterior (**a**) and lateral (**b**) chest radiographs

CT Images

Cardiovascular Angiography

15.1.3 Imaging Findings and Diagnosis

Chest radiograph showed increased pulmonary blood, right heart enlargement, the heart shadow was like a snowman shape (Fig. 15.1). CT angiography showed that the left and right pulmonary veins were not connected with left atrium and a small defect in the middle atrial septum. All the left and right pulmonary veins merged into a main trunk and ran upward to form vertical veins and merged into the innominate vein and superior vena cava and then entered to the right atrium (Fig. 15.2). Cardiovascular angiography also showed that all the pulmonary veins converge into a main trunk, ascending to form a vertical vein, converging into the innominate vein and superior vena cava and entering the right atrium (Fig. 15.3).

15.1.4 Management

- The patient underwent complete APVC correction plus repair of atrial septal defect surgery.

15.2 Discussion

Abnormal connection between a pulmonary vein and systemic vein will result in volume overload of the right heart, with a physiological effect similar to that of an ASD. All or part of the blood from the systemic venous and pulmonary circulation flows into the right atrium, forming mixed blood. Most of the blood enters the pulmonary circulation through the pulmonary artery, leading to increased blood flow in the pulmonary circulation, which is easy to form pulmonary hypertension. A portion of the blood enters the left heart through the patent foramen ovale or ventricular septal defect, and then enters the systemic circulation. Because it is mixed blood, blood oxygen content is low which causes cyanosis.

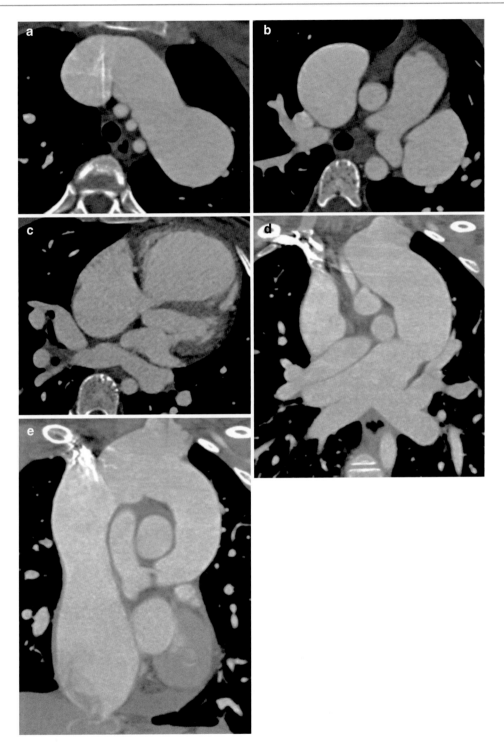

Fig. 15.2 CT findings of complete APVC. (**a**) Transverse axial view showed dilated abnormal draining veins in front of the three brachiocephalic arteries; (**b**) The pulmonary artery was dilated. The dilated abnormal vein was in the left of the pulmonary artery and the right of the aorta. (**c**) Transverse axial view showed enlarged right atrium and ventricle, relative small left atrium and ventricle, the pulmonary vein not connected with left atrium and a small defect in the middle atrial septum. (**d**) MIP showed that the left and right pulmonary veins merged into a main trunk and ran upward to form vertical veins. (**e**) MIP showed that the vertical veins merged into the innominate vein and superior vena cava and then entered the right atrium

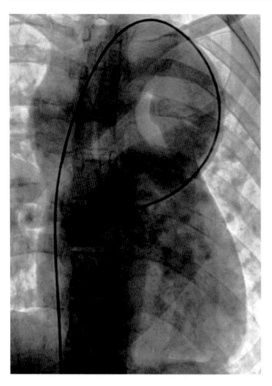

Fig. 15.3 Cardiovascular angiography of complete APVC. The left and right pulmonary veins converge into a main trunk, ascending to form a vertical vein, converging into the innominate vein and superior vena cava and entering the right atrium

Clinical symptoms mainly depend on the presence of pulmonary vein obstruction and the size of atrioventricular channel. Due to the stenosis of the pulmonary vein, the pulmonary vascular resistance increased, and left-to-right shunt will increase the pulmonary blood flow, leading to pulmonary hypertension, causing hypoxia and heart failure symptoms. For the surgeon, the main concerns are the presence of obstruction on the pulmonary venous and the location of abnormal connection of pulmonary venous (especially the relationship between the pulmonary venous confluence and the location of the left atrium), which are critical for the selection of surgical methods.

15.3 Current Technique Status and Applications of CT

CTA is recommended for the evaluation of partial anomalous pulmonary venous connection as first-line modality. Invasive cardiovascular angiography showed that pulmonary veins were usually recirculated, it is difficult to make an accurate diagnosis. It is useful for direct measurement of pressures, quantification of shunt magnitude, and measurement of pulmonary arterial resistance and responsiveness to pulmonary vasodilator therapy. CT images show one or more pulmonary veins connected directly to the vena cava or right atrium, either on one side or on both sides. The pulmonary veins in the heart were usually drawn into the vertical vein—left innominate vein—right superior vena cava—right atrium. Endocardial pulmonary veins are often drawn into the right atrium or coronary sinus. In sub-cardiac type, pulmonary veins often drain into the inferior lumen, portal vein, and hepatic vein. Multiplanar reconstruction and volumetric reconstruction can be used to show the stenosis of pulmonary veins. The indirect signs include the signs of pulmonary hypertension, the relative small left atrium and ventricle and other combined malformations. Lately, the new application of wide detector whole cardiac coverage CT increased the temporal resolution and decreased the radiation dose with low tube voltage.

15.4 Key Points

- APVC is a congenital cardiac malformation which refers to single or multiple pulmonary veins that are not connected to the anatomic left atrium, but directly into the systemic venous and right atrium.
- Cardiac CT examination may contribute to make a clear anatomic diagnosis.

Atrial Septal Defect

16

Yitong Yu and Bin Lu

Abstract

Atrial septal defects (ASDs) represent defects in the interatrial septum that allow left to right shunting. ASD is common, accounting for about 10–15% of congenital heart disease. The clinical consequences of an ASD are associated to the anatomic location of the defect, its size, and the presence or absence of other cardiac anomalies. ASDs are classified based on their anatomic location: primum ASD; secundum ASD; sinus venosus defect, in the wall between the left atrium and the superior vena cava or inferior vena cava; coronary sinus defect (unroofed coronary sinus defect) in the wall separating the coronary sinus from left atrium. Echocardiography is the first choice for the diagnosis of ASD. Magnetic resonance imaging can help to select cases with suspected associated defects such as partial anomalous pulmonary venous connection or patients in whom there are inconclusive echocardiographic findings. CT is one of the best methods for special types of ASD, such as coronary sinus defects or combined with ectopic pulmonary venous drainage. Surgical and transcatheter closure are the treatments for patients with indications.

16.1 Case of ASD

16.1.1 History

- An infant of 1 year and 11 months found a heart murmur by physical examination.
- The patient had no discomfort, denied syncope and hemoptysis.
- There was no significant difference in growth and intelligence between the patient and his peers.

Physical Examination
- Blood pressure: 130/74 mmHg; Breathing rate: 18/min
- Heart rate: 99 bpm without arrhythmia
- II–III systolic blowing murmur in the second and third intercostals at the left sternal border accompanied by a fixed split-second heart sound (S_2).
- Precordial bulge can be seen.

Electrocardiograph
Electrocardiogram shows sinus rhythm.

Laboratory
All laboratory tests showed negative results.

Y. Yu · B. Lu (✉)
Department of Radiology, Fuwai Hospital, Chinese Academy of Medical Sciences and Peking Union Medical College, Beijing, China

© Springer Nature Singapore Pte Ltd. 2020
Z.-y. Jin et al. (eds.), *Cardiac CT*, https://doi.org/10.1007/978-981-15-5305-9_16

16.1.2 Imaging Examination

Chest Radiograph

CT Images

Echocardiography

16.1.3 Imaging Findings and Diagnosis

The patient is a 1 year and 11 months old boy detected II–III systolic blowing murmur in the second and third intercostals at the left sternal border accompanied by a fixed split-second heart sound (S2). The increase in pulmonary vascularity, the prominent pulmonary trunk, and dilated central branches indicated left-to-right shunt (Fig. 16.1). Right atrium and right ventricle were enlarged reminded defect at the level of atrium (Fig. 16.2). Transthoracic echocardiogram found a defect in the wall between the left atrium and the inferior vena cava of 19 mm, with almost no stump in the posterior wall of atrium and the inferior vena cava constituting the defect bottom.

Left to right shunting across can be seen at the atrial septal defect. Right atrium and right ventricle enlarged and tricuspid inflow velocity (TVI) of 3 m/s (Fig. 16.3). CT confirmed this is a sinus venosus defect and excluded special types of ASD, such as coronary sinus defects, or combined with ectopic pulmonary venous drainage.

16.1.4 Management

- The patient underwent successful device closure of the defect.
- No murmurs and no increased pulmonary vascularity detected, prominent pulmonary trunk and dilated central pulmonary branches disappeared.
- The volume of the right atrium and ventricle were being followed up.

16.2 Discussion

ASD is a common congenital heart disease with clinical courses ranging from benign incidental finding on physical examination to complex

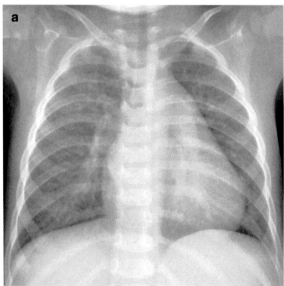 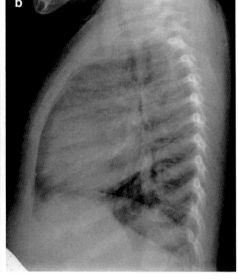

Fig. 16.1 Chest radiograph: Posterior-Anterior view (**a**) and left lateral view (**b**) shows lungs, pulmonary arteries, aorta, and heart. The increase in pulmonary vascularity extends to the periphery of the lung fields, the pulmonary trunk shows prominent and central branches appear dilated. The right atrium and ventricle were enlarged

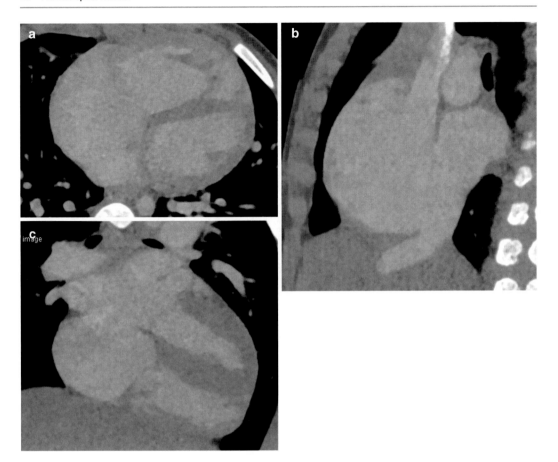

Fig. 16.2 Cardiac CT imaging: axial view (**a**), sagittal view (**b**), and coronal view (**c**) shows atrial septal defect. A sinus venosus defect which in the wall between the left atrium and the inferior vena cava was shown. Note the right atrial and the right ventricular enlargement (**a**)

lesions with significant intracardiac shunting and heart failure [1]. ASDs are classified as primum ASD, secundum ASD, sinus venosus defect, and coronary sinus defect. Primum ASDs account for 15–20% of ASDs. They develop when the septum primum does not fuse with the endocardial cushions. This results in a defect at the base of the interatrial septum that typically is associated with atrioventricular canal defects (e.g., anomalies of the atrioventricular valves and ventricular septal defects). Secundum ASD that is in the midportion of the atrial septum account for approximately 70% of all ASDs and generally present as an isolated defect. They are due to arrested growth of the secundum septum or excessive absorption of the primum septum resulting in an opening in the fossa ovalis. Sinus venosus defects have a high relation to partial

anomalous pulmonary venous return, and coronary sinus defects have a high relation to a persistent left superior vena cava.

The diagnosis of ASD is not difficult, but a refined diagnosis is required, such as the size of ASD position, the number of defects, the relationship with superior and inferior vena cava, aortic root, and left and right pulmonary veins. Small ASDs should be distinguished from patent foramen ovale which is less than 5 mm in diameter. Echocardiogram can detect the echo of the ovale fossa in two layers, with oblique gaps in the middle.

Echocardiogram is the tool of choice for diagnosis. Transthoracic echocardiogram (TTE) with color Doppler can show the jet of blood from the left atrium to the right atrium. If the ASD is not visualized on TTE, transesophageal

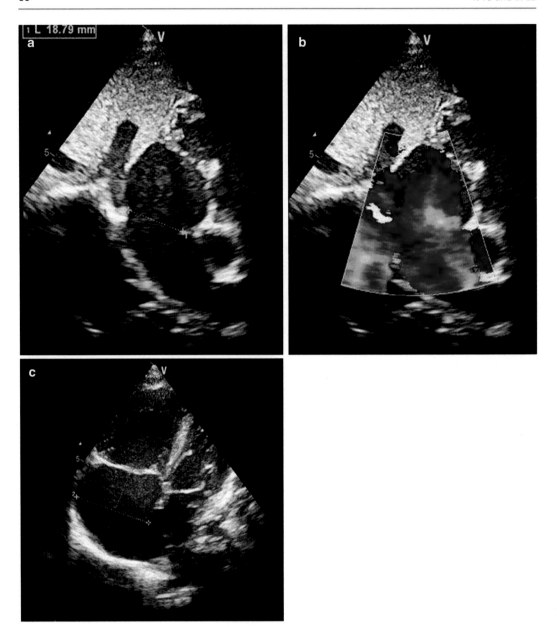

Fig. 16.3 Transthoracic echocardiogram showed ASD (sinus venosus defect). Subcostal view (**a**): a large defect in the wall between the left atrium and the inferior vena cava of 19 mm, with almost no stump in the posterior wall of atrium and the inferior vena cava constituting the defect bottom. Subcostal view (**b**): left to right shunting across the atrial septal defect. Apical four-chamber view (**c**): the right atrium and the right ventricle enlarged. Tricuspid inflow velocity (TVI) of 3 m/s

echocardiogram (TEE) may be required; it can also aid to size and determine concomitant abnormalities [2].

CT is required for preoperative screening for other malformations and excluded abnormal extracardiac structures.

ASD defects larger than 8 mm in diameter with significant left-to-right shunting may undergo spontaneous closure in childhood [3–5]. Persistent defects with pulmonary to systemic flow ratios (Qp/Qs) of >1.5 should be operated before school age or whenever a diagnosis is made if later [6]. Surgical closure was the preferred treatment until the 1990s and still the only treatment for large ASD defects [7]. For smaller defects, there were various devices for transcatheter closure of ASDs and it was an alternative to surgical treatment [8].

16.3 Current Technical Status and Applications of CT

Echocardiography is an excellent modality that is central to the diagnosis and treatment of ASDs. However, echocardiography has limited use in patients with poor acoustic windows, especially in obesity, chest wall deformities, as well as chronic obstructive pulmonary diseases. What is more, prior interventions and metallic devices increase the difficulty of the examination [9]. A research reported that the echocardiography and CT have their own advantages and disadvantages, with diagnostic accuracy both over 90%. Echocardiography has relatively high sensitivity in detecting intracardiac structure abnormalities, but less sensitivity than 64-slice spiral CT method when diagnosing the extracardiac structural abnormalities. Hence, the combination of the two methods is recommended to improve the diagnosis of congenital heart disease [10].

CT has several advantages and is important in the assessment of congenital heart disease. First, CT is widely available and required a short time for image acquisition. Second, CT has an advantage in imaging small structures (e.g., coronary artery) with its high isovolumetric spatial resolution (on the order of 0.25 mm^3 voxel volume). What is more, the dynamic evaluation can be obtained with the good temporal resolution of CT. In addition, the post-processing of CT images with multiplanar reconstruction and volume reconstruction, wide field of view without acoustic window limitations make CT superior in the evaluation of extracardiac structures than echocardiography. Recently, 3D printouts can be acquired from 3D images produced by CT volume reconstruction. This is promising and favorable in preoperative planning, shorter surgical time, and is helpful in conformation or even improvement of the surgery options, especially for complex congenital heart disease [11, 12].

For shunt lesions, CT is a suboptimal choice when echocardiography fails to exam and cardiac MR imaging is infeasible or restricted by artifacts. CT is one of the best methods for special types of ASD, such as coronary sinus defects or combined with ectopic pulmonary venous drainage and persistent left superior vena cava. The anatomic location, size, and coexistence of other cardiac anomalies are crucial to the results of repair [7].

Meanwhile, there are some disadvantages of CT. CT has ionizing radiation, which may result in a theoretic risk of cancer, especially in young and female in serial surveillance imaging. Nowadays, many proposals have been suggested to reduce CT radiation dose. Omitting the test bolus or bolus tracking scan optimize cardiac CT radiation dose which can have a relevant share of radiation exposure, especially in neonates [13]. In addition, patients with renal dysfunction, especially with a history of acute renal insufficiency and repeated contrast injections should be cautious of the contrast-induced nephrotoxicity; however, the low incidence (0.85%) has been shown in recent studies [14].

In conclusion, CT is an important noninvasive imaging modality for the evaluation of ASD, particularly useful for the assessment of cardiac and extracardiac anatomy and function in patients with suboptimal echocardiography and infeasible or technically restricted MR imaging. CT is also critical to evaluate small structures and make preoperative planning [9].

16.4 Key Points

- Atrial septal defect (ASD) is common, accounting for about 10–15% of congenital heart disease. The clinical consequences of an ASD are related to the anatomic location and size of the defect, and the presence or absence of other cardiac anomalies.
- CT is an important noninvasive imaging modality for the evaluation of ASD, particularly useful for the assessment of cardiac and extracardiac anatomy and function.

References

1. Hari P, Pai RG, Varadarajan P. Echocardiographic evaluation of patent foramen ovale and atrial septal defect. Echocardiography. 2015;32(Suppl 2):S110–24.
2. Thompson E. Atrial septal defect. JAAPA. 2013;26(6):53–4.
3. Radzik D, Davignon A, Van Doesberg N, et al. Spontaneous closure of an atrial septal defect. J Am Med Assoc. 1966;196:137–9.
4. Cayler GG. Spontaneous functional closure of symptomatic atrial septal defects. New Eng J Med. 1967;276:65–70.
5. Grech V. Atrial septal defect in Malta. J Paediatr Child Health. 1999;35:190–5.
6. Kirklin JW, Barratt-Bouyes G. Cardiac surgery. 2nd ed. New York: Churchill Livingstone; 1999. p. 609–44.
7. Bloomingdale R, Ashraf S, Cardozo S. Atrial septal defect repair gone wrong. Echocardiography. 2017;34:315–6.
8. Ebeid MR. Percutaneous catheter closure of secundum atrial septal defects: a review. J Invasive Cardiol. 2002;14:25–31.
9. Ranganath P, Singh S, Abbara S, et al. Computed tomography in adult congenital heart disease. Radiol Clin N Am. 2019;57(1):85–111.
10. Mei M, Nie J, Yang ZS, et al. Comparison of echocardiography and 64-slice spiral computed tomography in the diagnosis of congenital heart disease in children. J Cell Biochem. 2019;120(3):3969–77.
11. Han F, Co-Vu J, Lopez-Colon D, et al. Impact of 3D printouts in optimizing surgical results for complex congenital heart disease. World J Pediatr Congenit Heart Surg. 2019;10(5):533–8.
12. Xu JJ, Luo YJ, Wang JH, et al. Patient-specific three-dimensional printed heart models benefit preoperative planning for complex congenital heart disease. World J Pediatr. 2019;15(3):246–54.
13. Schindler P, Kehl HG, Wildgruber M, et al. Cardiac CT in the preoperative diagnostics of neonates with congenital heart disease: radiation dose optimization by omitting test bolus or bolus tracking. Acad Radiol. 2019. pii: S1076-6332(19)30368-X.
14. Krause TM, Ukhanova M, Lee Revere F, et al. Risk predictors for postcontrast acute kidney injury. J Am Coll Radiol. 2018;15(11):1547–52.

Ventricular Septal Defect

17

Xinshuang Ren and Bin Lu

Abstract

Ventricular septal defects (VSD) was a common congenital cardiac abnormality with defects in the interventricular septum results in a hemodynamic communication between the right and left ventricles. It is considered the most common congenital cardiac disease diagnosed in children and the second most common in adults. It accounts for approximately 40% of congenital heart disease. Clinical presentation varies depending on the defect size and degree of the shunt. The diagnosis can be accomplished by echocardiography or CTA with ECG-gating with direct visualization of the septal defect. Surgical and transcatheter closure of the defect were commonly used, while defect closure in patients with raised pulmonary vascular resistance can result in substantial morbidity and mortality.

17.1 Case of VSD

17.1.1 History

- Four-months-old male infant cough for several days and systolic murmur was heard over the left sternal border during physical examination.
- X-ray and CT examination were suggested to observe cardiac structure.

Physical Examination
- Blood pressure: 90/60 mmHg; Breathing rate: 30/min
- Heart rate: 155 bpm without arrhythmia
- 3/6 grade systolic murmur heard on the left border of sternum.

Laboratory
Serum myocardial enzyme spectrum showed negative results.

17.1.2 Imaging Examination

X-ray Images

CT Images

X. Ren · B. Lu (✉)
Department of Radiology, Fuwai Hospital, Chinese Academy of Medical Sciences and Peking Union Medical College, Beijing, China

© Springer Nature Singapore Pte Ltd. 2020
Z.-y. Jin et al. (eds.), *Cardiac CT*, https://doi.org/10.1007/978-981-15-5305-9_17

17.1.3 Imaging Findings and Diagnosis

The X-ray image demonstrates prominent pulmonary vasculature (active congestion) without pleural effusions or convincing consolidation and cardiomegaly with prominence of the main pulmonary trunk.

CT images demonstrate subarterial ventricular septal defect. Enlarged left ventricle and dilated pulmonary trunk was shown (Figs. 17.1 and 17.2).

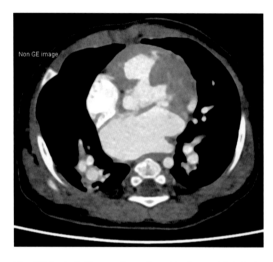

Fig. 17.1 Axial image showed ventricular septal defect

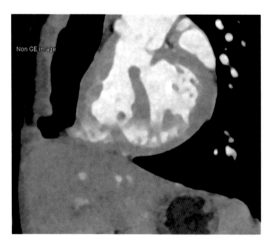

Fig. 17.2 Reconstructed image showed ventricular septal defect

17.1.4 Management

- Surgical closure of VSD
- Out-patient follow-up observations

17.2 Discussion

VSD is one of the most common congenital heart malformations, accounting for up to 40% of all congenital heart anomalies. The frequency of this defect varies with age since many tiny muscular defects reported by highly sensitive color Doppler echocardiography shortly disappear during the first year of life [1].

VSD is classified into three types according to defect location: perimembranous, infundibular, and muscular VSD. The clinical consequences of a VSD is related to the amount and direction of interventricular shunting. The size of the defect and relative resistances of pulmonary vascular beds determine the amount of interventricular amount. Neonatus with VSD might experiences minimal left-to-right shunting due to high pulmonary vascular resistance, while the shunting rises and the patient develops symptoms as pulmonary vascular resistance falls. Excessive pulmonary blood flow will result in increased pulmonary vascular resistance, the amount of interventricular left-to-right shunting could decrease and eventually lead to right-to-left shunting causing cyanosis and Eisenmenger's syndrome.

Typical X-ray image shows prominent pulmonary vasculature and enlarged heart, especially the enlargement of the left ventricle. CT images show the defect directly and contrast agents connect between the left and right ventricles [2]. Left and right ventricles and left atrium are enlarged. Dilated pulmonary artery can also be seen to reflect pulmonary hypertension.

Patch closure of a ventricular septal defect through sternotomy was commonly used in the past 50 years. Transcatheter techniques for closure of ventricular septal defects have been developed in the few decades. Surgical closure in patients developed pulmonary hypertension can result in substantial morbidity and mortality due to right ventricular failure caused by increased pulmonary blood flow and right ventricle pressure. Supportive treatment is appropriate for individuals with Eisenmenger's syndrome.

17.3 Current Technical Status and Applications of CT

CT is an important imaging modality in the evaluation of congenital heart disease with three-dimensional reconstruction and rapid prototyping technology of multislice spiral computed tomography angiography (CTA). CT also requires no sedation and has shorter scan duration. CT can also provide detailed information of extracardiac abnormalities [3].

CT images show direct visualization of the defect with a high sensitivity and specificity. Size measurements can be comprehensively obtained with short diameter, normalized area, and relative area, which is hardly obtained by two-dimensional echocardiography. Patients with VSD might combine with other congenital heart disease requiring additional imaging evaluation beyond echocardiography [4]. CT images are able to simultaneously assess associated anomalies with high spatial and temporal resolution beyond the echocardiographic window.

17.4 Key Points

- Ventricular septal defect accounts for up to 40% of all congenital cardiac anomalies.
- The chest radiograph can be normal with a small VSD. Larger VSDs showed prominent pulmonary vasculature and enlarged heart, especially the enlargement of left ventricle in X-ray image.
- CT images show the defect directly. Left and right ventricles and left atrium are enlarged, features of pulmonary arterial hypertension, pulmonary edema, pleural effusion.

References

1. Barboza JM, Dajani NK, Glenn LG, et al. Prenatal diagnosis of congenital cardiac anomalies: a practical approach using two basic views. Radiographics. 2002;22(5):1125–37.
2. Goo HW, Park IS, Ko JK et al. CT of congenital heart disease: normal anatomy and typical pathologic conditions. Radiographics. 2003;23 Spec No: S147-65.
3. Nau D, Wuest W, Rompel O, et al. Evaluation of ventricular septal defects using high pitch computed tomography angiography of the chest in children with complex congenital heart defects below one year of age. J Cardiovasc Comput Tomogr. 2019;13(4):226–33.
4. Penny DJ, Vick GW III. ventricular septal defect. Lancet. 2011;377(9771):1103–12.

Double Outlet Right Ventricle

18

Zhihui Hou and Bin Lu

Abstract

Double outlet right ventricle (DORV) is a complex congenital heart disease with variable morphology and hemodynamics. Imaging plays an important role in the determination and characterization of outflow tract. Computed tomography (CT) with advanced three-dimensional post-processing techniques is invaluable in defining the anatomy of DORV with simultaneous assessment of associated anomalies.

18.1 Case of DORV

18.1.1 History

- Eleven-months-old boy.
- Prenatal ultrasound found congenital heart disease.
- Eleven months after birth, he did cardiac CT examination in order to identify anatomic abnormalities of the heart.

Physical Examination

- Blood pressure: 89/77 mmHg; Breathing rate: 21/min.
- Heart rate: 121 bpm without arrhythmia.
- 2/6 grade systolic murmurs are audible in sternum left edge.

Electrocardiograph

Abnormal P wave, biventricular hypertrophy.

Laboratory

- Red blood cell count elevated (6.24×10^{12}/L)
- C-reactive protein elevated (7.31 mg/L)

18.1.2 Imaging Examination

X-ray Exam

CT Images

18.1.3 Imaging Findings and Diagnosis

The chest X-ray radiograph showed a small amount of blood in both lungs and an enlarged right ventricle, which was very similar to the tetralogy of Fallot (Fig. 18.1). CT angiography suggested that both aorta and pulmonary artery originated from the right ventricle (Fig. 18.2), the right ventricle was enlarged, the ventricular septal defect was close to the aortic valve (Fig. 18.3), and pulmonary

Z. Hou · B. Lu (✉)
Department of Radiology, Fuwai Hospital, Chinese Academy of Medical Sciences and Peking Union Medical College, Beijing, China

© Springer Nature Singapore Pte Ltd. 2020
Z.-y. Jin et al. (eds.), *Cardiac CT*, https://doi.org/10.1007/978-981-15-5305-9_18

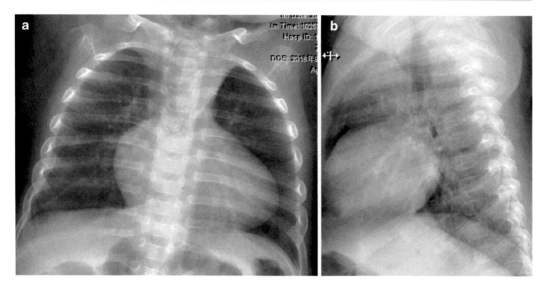

Fig. 18.1 Chest X-ray. Anteroposterior (**a**) and lateral (**b**) radiographs

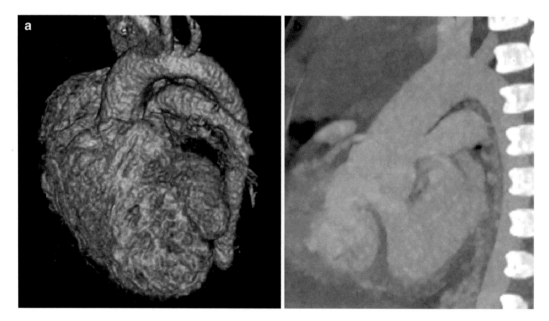

Fig. 18.2 Three-dimensional volume-rendered images of CT angiography (**a**) and reformatted CT angiography image (**b**) show both aorta and pulmonary artery arising entirely from the right ventricle

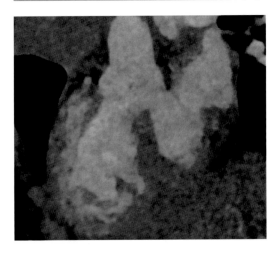

Fig. 18.3 Reformatted CT angiography image shows subaortic ventricular septal defect

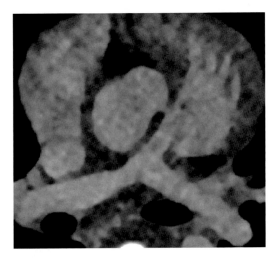

Fig. 18.4 Axial CT angiography image shows the presence of pulmonary stenosis

artery stenosis was combined (Fig. 18.4). Finally, it was diagnosed as DORV (Tetralogy of Fallot-type variant) for subaortic ventricular septal defect (VSD) with pulmonary stenosis (PS).

18.1.4 Management

- Surgical repairs: Blalock–Taussig shunt, bidirectional Glenn shunt, total cavopulmonary connection, and Fontan circulation.

18.2 Discussion

DORV is a complex congenital heart disease, wherein both the pulmonary artery and aorta are committed either >50% or completely to the right ventricle (RV). The classification of DORV is based on the location of VSD and the presence/absence of PS, with the common subtypes of DORV being as follows: (1) tetralogy of Fallot-type variant (subaortic VSD with PS); (2) transposition of great arteries-type variant (subpulmonary VSD without PS): Taussig–Bing anomaly; (3) VSD-type variant (subaortic VSD without PS); and (4) univentricular heart-type variant (DORV with mitral atresia, unbalanced atrioventricular canal, or presence of severe hypoplasia of one of the ventricular sinuses) [1, 2]. VSD location affects the physiology and influences the surgical management significantly. The VSD may be as follows: (1) subaortic; (2) subpulmonary; (3) noncommitted; and (4) doubly committed in relation to the semilunar valves.

Echocardiography often constitutes the first-line of diagnostic imaging. Catheter angiography, formerly considered the reference standard of diagnosis, is an invasive procedure with an inherent risk of complications [3]. Magnetic resonance imaging (MRI) is a promising imaging tool because of the lack of radiation risks and the availability of accurate functional assessment. However, it has several inherent disadvantages including long acquisition times, need for sedation or general anesthesia, poor spatial resolution, and limited availability [4]. Current-generation CT scanners can provide excellent image quality with high spatial and temporal resolution. Moreover, recent technical advancements have resulted in reduction of the scanning time as well as radiation dose in pediatric patients [5].

18.3 Current Technical Status and Applications of CT

CT generally requires no sedation, and thus allows for detailed evaluation of extracardiac abnormalities. The CT data set can also be used in 3D printing, which can be useful in planning and predicting successful surgical outcomes. A highly important surgical determinant is the routability of the VSD. The location of the VSD depends on its relationship to the semilunar valve and the orientation of the outlet septum. The location of the VSD in relation to the tricuspid annulus is also important [6]. In subaortic VSD, repair is carried out by creating an intraventricular tunnel. Arterial switch operation with the creation of aorta to ventricular tunnel is preferred in subpulmonary VSD with right ventricular outflow obstruction. Doubly committed VSD also involves tunnel repair, whereas noncommitted VSD requires complex biventricular repair if the ventricles are of an adequate size [7]. CT can provide other information of associated anomalies, including sizing of ventricles, aortic anomalies, pulmonary arterial anomalies, anomalous systemic and pulmonary venous drainage, and coronary arterial anomalies.

18.4 Key Points

- The classification of DORV is primarily based on the location of VSD and the presence/absence of PS.
- CT seems a well-suited choice in the imaging evaluation of DORV. It can provide information on the location of the VSD and routability and other information on associated anomalies.

References

1. Freedon R, Smallhorn J. Double outlet right ventricle. In: Freedon R, Benson L, Smallhorn J, editors. Neonatal heart disease. 1st ed. London: Springer; 1992. p. 453–70.
2. Frank L, Dillman JR, Parish V, et al. Cardiovascular MR imaging of conotruncal anomalies. Radiographics. 2010;30:1069–94.
3. Vitiello R, McCrindle BW, Nykanen D, et al. Complications associated with pediatric cardiac catheterization. J Am Coll Cardiol. 1998;32:1433–40.
4. Tangcharoen T, Bell A, Hegde S, et al. Detection of coronary artery anomalies in infants and young children with congenital heart disease by using MR imaging. Radiology. 2011;259:240–7.
5. Shi K, Yang ZG, Chen J, et al. Assessment of double outlet right ventricle associated with multiple malformations in pediatric patients using retrospective ECG-gated dual-source computed tomography. PLoS One. 2015;10:e0130987.
6. Yim D, Dragulescu A, Ide H, et al. Essential modifiers of double outlet right ventricle: revisit with endocardial surface images and 3-dimensional print models. Circ Cardiovasc Imaging. 2018;11:e006891.
7. Cetta F, Boston US, Dearani JA, et al. Double outlet right ventricle: opinions regarding management. Curr Treat Options Cardiovasc Med. 2005;7:385–90.

Patent Ductus Arteriosus

19

Na Zhao, Yang Gao, and Bin Lu

Abstract

Patent ductus arteriosus (PDA) is the continuous connection between the pulmonary artery and aortic after birth, resulting in an abnormal shunt through ductus. It is one of the most common congenital heart diseases, which can exist alone or can be combined with other congenital cardiac malformations. The diagnosis can be accomplished by noninvasive imaging examination. However, more details need to be evaluated before clinical decision-making. In this chapter, based on a typical case, we will make a systematic understanding of PDA and discuss the role of CT in the diagnosis and treatment of PDA.

19.1 Case of PDA

19.1.1 History

- A 52-year-old female patient was identified with a cardiac murmur detected by a routine physical examination in more than 20 years ago.

- Dyspnea on exertion and occasional precordial pain occurred without edema of lower limbs in the last 3 years.

Physical Examination
- Auscultation: a "machinery" murmur was heard at the second interspace to the left sternum through the entire cardiac cycle.

19.1.2 Imaging Examination

Echocardiogram
Echocardiogram revealed a patent ductus arteriosus extended between the left pulmonary artery and descending thoracic aortic isthmus. The inner diameter of the patent ductus was about 9 mm. And a left-to-right shunting through the ductus arteriosus was detected.

X-Ray (Fig. 19.1)

CT Images (Fig. 19.2)

Cardiac Angiography (Fig. 19.3)

19.1.3 Imaging Findings and Diagnosis

The CTA images, echocardiography, and aortic angiography manifested the patent ductus arteriosus connecting the proximal descending aorta

N. Zhao · Y. Gao · B. Lu (✉)
Department of Radiology, Fuwai Hospital, Chinese Academy of Medical Sciences and Peking Union Medical College, Beijing, China

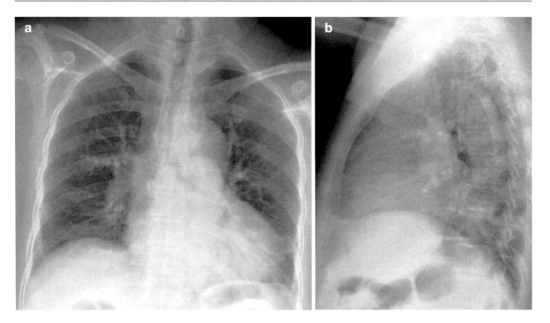

Fig. 19.1 The pulmonary artery was prominent. And pulmonary vessels in the lungs were enlarged, indicating the increased pulmonary blood flow. In the anteroposterior (**a**) and left lateral (**b**) projection, the apex was low and downward due to the left ventricular enlargement. The cardiothoracic ratio was 0.60

and main pulmonary artery. Left-to-right shunting through the ductus arteriosus could be detected by echocardiography and aortic angiography. The apex was low and downward due to the left ventricular enlargement (Fig. 19.1). PDA can be clearly diagnosed with a comprehensive analysis of the signs above (Figs. 19.2 and 19.3).

19.1.4 Management

The patient underwent patent ductus arteriosus occlusive operation. A 16/14 mm ductal occlusive device was implanted. When the left-to-right shunt through ductus disappeared during the procedure, the occlusive device was successfully released.

19.2 Discussion

The ductus arteriosus is a fetal vascular structure between the proximal descending aorta and the main pulmonary artery, which normally closes spontaneously after birth. The patent ductus arteriosus (PDA) is the neonatal persistence of the essential conduit. It has been reported that the incidence of PDA is 1 in 2000 term newborns and the female-to-male ratio is about 2:1 [1, 2]. This accounts for 5–10% of all congenital heart disease.

The lungs of the fetus have no ventilation functions and pulmonary circulation resistance is high. The blood from right ventricle mainly flows into the descending aorta through the ductus arteriosus in fetal period. Then the pulmonary circula-

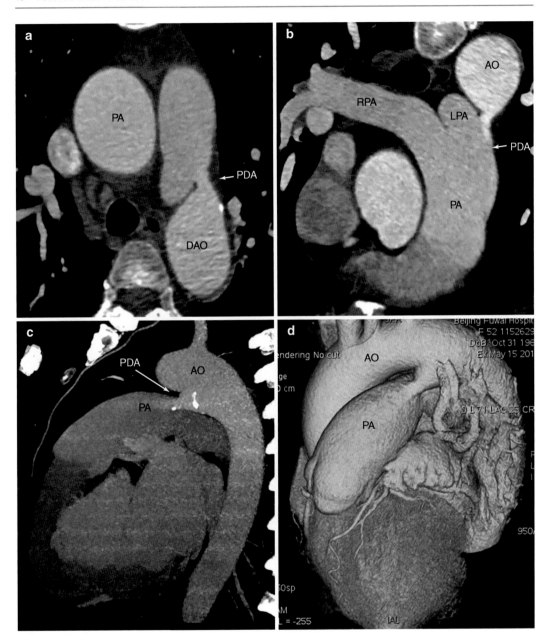

Fig. 19.2 (**a**, **e**, axial view; **b**, **c**, MPR; **d**, VR; **f**, **g**, **h**, CPR) The axial view (**a**), multi-planar reformation (**b**, **c**) and volume rendering (**d**) showed the patent ductus arteriosus extended between proximal descending aorta and pulmonary artery. (**e**) Axial view also manifested the enlargement of the left atrium and ventricular. Curved planar reconstruction (**f**, **g**, **h**) showed unobstructed lumens of LAD, RCA, and LCX

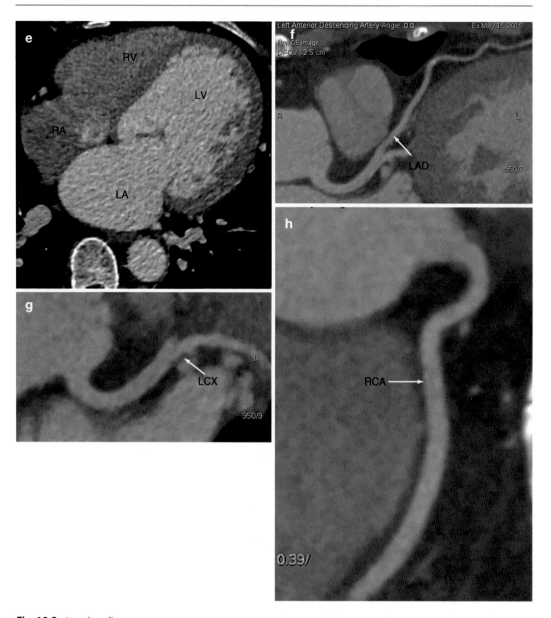

Fig. 19.2 (continued)

tion resistance decreased being lower than aortic pressure as the lungs inflate after birth, and the blood flows directly into pulmonary arteries from right ventricle. When the ductus persists, the shunting from the aorta to the pulmonary artery (the left-to-right shunt) can lead to a series of hemodynamic and pathophysiological changes such as pulmonary over-circulation, a progressive

increase in pulmonary vascular resistance and systemic hypoperfusion. When pulmonary vascular resistance exceeds the systemic vascular resistance, ductal shunting reverses causing cyanosis.

The symptoms of PDA patients vary a lot, depending on the shunt, pulmonary vascular resistance, age, and complicated with other malformations. There may be no obvious clinical

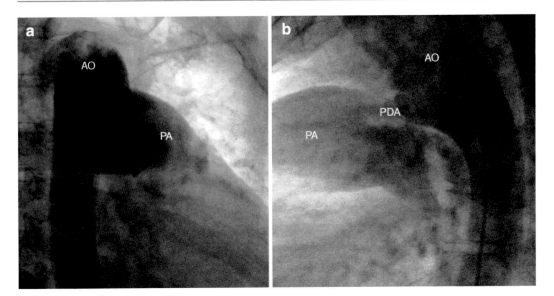

Fig. 19.3 Aortic angiogram showed the pulmonary arteries imaging could be immediately obtained after aortic imaging indicating the left-to-right shunting (**a**). In lateral projection (**b**), the ductus arteriosus was showed which connected the proximal descending aorta and the main pulmonary artery

symptoms in patients with small shunts. However, most patients may have complaints of palpitations, shortness of breath, fatigue, chest pain, recurrent respiratory tract infection, and stunting of growth in infancy. In the physical examination, the hallmark indicator is a continuous "machinery" murmur, located at the left margin of the sternum between the second and third interspaces. In the patient with a large ductus arteriosus, ECG may demonstrate sinus tachycardia or atrial fibrillation, left ventricular hypertrophy, and left atrial enlargement [3].

The typical imaging feature is the patent arteriosus extending between descending aorta and the main pulmonary artery closely to the root of left pulmonary vessel. And the echocardiogram is still the procedure of choice to make a diagnosis of PDA and then do many evaluations. The M-mode echocardiography can be used to measure the cardiac chamber sizes and evaluate left ventricular systolic function. And the degree of ductal shunting can be estimated sensitively and effectively by color Doppler. Depending on the amount of shunting, the chest film may be normal or demonstrate cardiomegaly with an enlarged

pulmonary artery. Enhanced CT examination could show the vascular connectivity between the proximal descending aortic and the distal main pulmonary artery. The axial view, volume reconstruction, and sagittal MPR reconstruction can clearly manifest the position of aortic and pulmonary artery, as well as the position, shape, and size of ductus arteriosus. In addition, CT can be used to identify and evaluate the development status of aorta and pulmonary artery, calcification of ductus arteriosus and other cardiac defects.

19.3 Current Technical Status and Applications of CT

The diagnosis and management decisions of PDA can be accomplished by echocardiography alone. However, the abnormalities beyond the sonographic window, complex three-dimensional lesions, and detailed functional information require additional imaging [4]. CT can be used to provide the information above and identify and evaluate other associated cardiac malformations. Nowadays, 3D imaging derived from CT is widely used to improve understanding of complex anatomy [5, 6]. Besides, for patients over 50 years old, it is necessary to rule out the possibility of coronary heart disease before operation. ECG-gated CT scan can make a definite diagnosis of coronary artery lesions and reduce unnecessary invasive coronary angiography. It not only saves the economic cost but also avoids the injury.

19.4   Key Points

- The patent ductus arteriosus (PDA) is a vascular structure that connects the proximal descending aorta to the roof of the main pulmonary artery near the origin of the left branch pulmonary artery.
- The diagnosis and management decisions of PDA can be simply accomplished by noninvasive imaging examination.
- CT provides the information beyond intracardiac structure for a comprehensive evaluation before treatment.

References

1. Carlgren LE. The incidence of congenital heart disease in children born in Gothenburg 1941–1950. Br Heart J. 1959;21:40–50.
2. Mitchell SC, Korones SB, Berendes HW. Congenital heart disease in 56,109 births: incidence and natural history. Circulation. 1971;43:323–32.
3. Schneider DJ, Moore JW. Patent ductus arteriosus. Circulation. 2006;114(17):1873–82. https://doi.org/10.1161/circulationaha.105.592063. PMID:17060397.
4. Chan FP, Hanneman K. Computed tomography and magnetic resonance imaging in neonates with congenital cardiovascular disease. Semin Ultrasound CT MR. 2015;36(2):146–60. https://doi.org/10.1053/j.sult.2015.01.006.PMID:26001944.
5. Kasprzak JD, Witowski J, Pawlowski J, et al. Percutaneous patent ductus arteriosus closure using intraprocedural mixed reality visualization of 3D computed tomography angiography data: first-in-man experience. Eur Heart J Cardiovasc Imaging. 2019;20(7):839. https://doi.org/10.1093/ehjci/jez008. PMID:31220228.
6. Saunders AB, Doocy KR, Birch SA. A pictorial view of the three-dimensional representation and comparative two-dimensional image orientation derived from computed tomography angiography in a dog with a patent ductus arteriosus. J Vet Cardiol. 2019;2019(21):34–40. https://doi.org/10.1016/j.jvc.2018.09.004.PMID:30797443.

Tetralogy of Fallot (TOF)

20

Wei-hua Yin and Bin Lu

Abstract

Tetralogy of Fallot (TOF) is a cyanotic congenital heart disorder that encompasses four anatomic abnormalities: overriding aorta, ventricular septal defect (VSD), right ventricular hypertrophy, and right ventricular (RV) outflow obstruction. The prevalence of TOF is approximately 4–5 per 10,000 live births in the United States. This disorder accounts for approximately 7–10% of cases of congenital heart disease requiring surgical intervention in the first year of life. Echocardiography is used to make the diagnosis of TOF generally. Electrocardiogram, CT, and chest radiography are often performed during the evaluation of TOF. Cardiac catheterization is sometimes used to further figure hemodynamic changes. Associated intracardiac and extracardiac anomalies and potential surgical palliations encountered must be taken into consideration when the diagnosis of TOF is made. Multidetector cardiac computed tomography (MDCT) has become a valuable modality in evaluating the complex anatomic disorders with its superior spatial and temporal resolution.

20.1 Case of TOF

20.1.1 History

- A 4-year-old boy found heart murmur for 5 months.

Physical Examination
- Blood pressure: 85/55mmHg; Breathing rate: 23/min.
- Heart rate: 150 bpm without arrhythmia.
- 3/6 grade systolic murmurs are audible in the left intercostal 3–4 region.

Electrocardiograph
Standard 12-lead electrocardiograph (ECG) revealed normal.

Laboratory
Oxygen saturation showed reduced oxygen partial pressure, hemoglobin and increased CO_2 partial pressure.

20.1.2 Imaging Examination

An X-ray (Fig. 20.1), cardiac CT (Fig. 20.3) combined with echocardiography (Fig. 20.2) were requested to investigate the intracardiac and extracardiac anomalies.

X-ray

W.-h. Yin · B. Lu (✉)
Department of Radiology, Fuwai Hospital, Chinese Academy of Medical Sciences and Peking Union Medical College, Beijing, China

© Springer Nature Singapore Pte Ltd. 2020
Z.-y. Jin et al. (eds.), *Cardiac CT*, https://doi.org/10.1007/978-981-15-5305-9_20

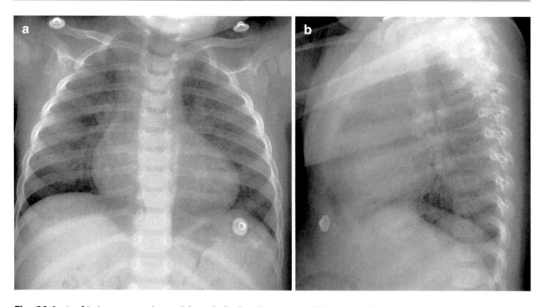

Fig. 20.1 (**a**, **b**) Anteroposterior and lateral display demonstrated less lung blood, pulmonary artery depression, enlargement of right atrial and ventricular

Echocardiography

CT Images

20.1.3 Imaging Findings and Diagnosis

The chest film can be used firstly for evaluation of lung and pulmonary vessels of TOF patients (Fig. 20.1). Cardiac CTA images results showed perimembranous ventricular septal defect (about 10 mm), the overriding aorta in continuity with mitral and tricuspid valves (40%), pulmonary valve thickening and adhesion, and pulmonary valve ring diameter is about 10 mm, severe right ventricular outflow tract obstruction, good pulmonary development, and right ventricular hypertrophy (Figs. 20.2 and 20.3).

Pulmonary arteries—The size and anatomy of the main pulmonary artery, and the proximal branch pulmonary arteries can also be assessed in cardiac CT.

Coronary arteries—The coronary anatomy is defined by CTA in patients with TOF.

20.1.4 Management

Most patients with TOF underwent intracardiac repair as their initial intervention by 1 year of age (typically before 6 months of age) [1]. A small minority of infants require palliative shunts or ductal stents prior to surgical repair. Shunts or stents may be necessary due to severe right ventricular outflow tract (RVOT) obstruction or, less commonly, medically refractory hypercyanotic ("tet") spells. Shunts or stents may also be used in infants who are not initially acceptable candidates for intracardiac repair due to hypoplastic pulmonary arteries (PAs), coronary artery anatomy, or prematurity.

Palliative intervention—A small subset of patients with TOF require early surgical or transcatheter palliative intervention before complete repair is performed.

20.2　Discussion

TOF is a complex congenital heart disease common in children, accounting for 10% of all congenital heart diseases. Accurate assessment of preoperative imaging is important for this surgical approach. The first choice for examination is echocardiography (UCG), but UCG cannot accurately assess the limitations of extracardiac vascular malformations, airway malformations,

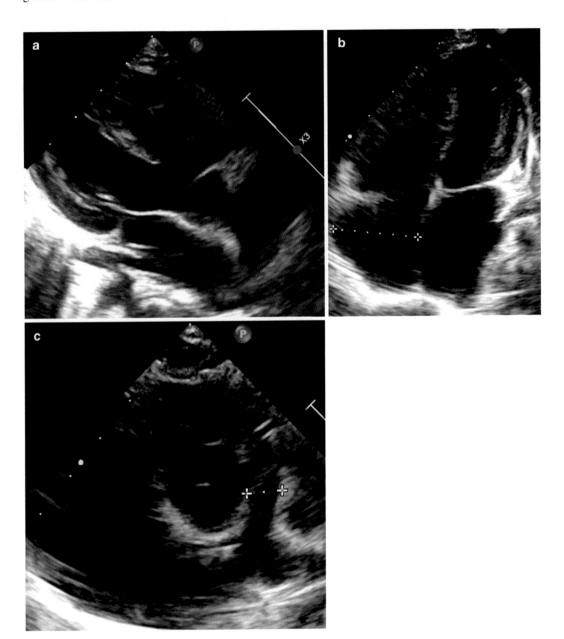

Fig. 20.2 Echocardiography showed that perimembranous ventricular septal defect (**a**), the overriding aorta in continuity with both the mitral and tricuspid valves (**a**), Right enlargement of right atrial and ventricular (**b**), ventricular hypertrophy. Pulmonary valve ring diameter is about 10 mm (**c**), and pulmonary valve thickening, adhesion and highly stenosis (**d**)

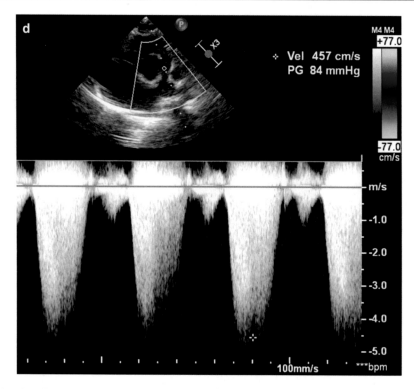

Fig. 20.2 (continued)

and vascular branches of the body's lungs. The diagnostic accuracy is also affected by the operator's dual skill level. CT has a very high temporal and spatial resolution and is widely distributed before surgery for cardiac and macrovascular diseases. It has become the primary screening tool for complex congenital heart disease.

TOF is a cyanotic congenital heart disorder that encompasses four anatomic features: overriding aorta, ventricular septal defect (VSD), right ventricular hypertrophy, and right ventricular (RV) outflow obstruction. The prevalence of TOF is approximately 4–5 per 10,000 live births in the United States [2, 3]. This disorder accounts for approximately 7–10% of cases of congenital heart disease requiring surgical intervention in the first year of life.

Echocardiography is used to make the diagnosis of TOF generally. Electrocardiogram, CT, and chest radiography are often performed during the evaluation of TOF. Cardiac catheterization is sometimes used to further figure hemodynamic changes. Associated intracardiac and extracardiac anomalies and potential surgical palliations encountered must be taken into consideration when the diagnosis of TOF was made. Multidetector cardiac computed tomography (MDCT) has become a valuable modality in evaluating the complex anatomic disorders with its superior spatial and temporal resolution.

Conclusively, MDCT is a safe, reliable, and low-cost diagnostic imaging modality, which offers accurate anatomic assessment for the complex spectrum of TOF.

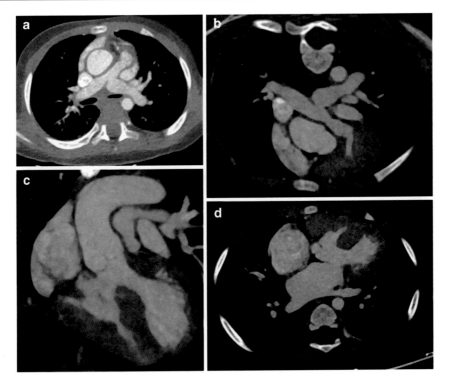

Fig. 20.3 Cardiac CT imaging: Pulmonary valve thickening and adhesion, and pulmonary valve ring diameter is about 10 mm (**a**). Severe right ventricular outflow tract obstruction, good pulmonary development (**b**). The overriding aorta in continuity with mitral and tricuspid valves (**c**), perimembranous ventricular septal defect and right ventricular hypertrophy (**d**)

20.3 Current Technical Status and Applications of CT

Although cardiac catheterization has advantages for accurate diagnosis, Cardiac Computed Tomographic (CT) scan technology has showed a complementary role for these patients. CT has gradually replaced angiography in the diagnosis of TOF. CT shows that cardiovascular disease can achieve approximate pathological anatomy from three-dimensional images, and has obvious advantages for complex congenital diseases. In addition, CT is superior to ultrasound in extracardiac large vessel anatomic deformity. Patients with TOF often have abnormal coronary origin and distribution. If these abnormal origins or coronary trunks and branches bypassed the right ventricular outflow tract, they are easily damaged during surgery. It will lead to myocardial ischemia or cause death. Ultrasound can only show the opening of the coronary artery, and the detection rate of coronary anomalies is very low.

In the past, ultrasound and invasive cardiovascular angiography were mainly used for the examination of congenital heart disease. Ultrasound has become the first choice and basic examination method with its advantages of noninvasive and simple. It shows great advantages in intracardiac malformation. For extracardiac pulmonary artery abnormalities, it is affected by many factors, and its display and diagnosis rate are low. CT for the detection rate of accompanying extracardiac malformation was significantly higher than that of ultrasound in TOF patients. Invasive cardiovascular angiography has become the gold standard for the diagnosis of congenital heart disease, but it is an invasive examination, complicated operation procedural, too much radiation dose, high examination cost, and is not suitable for routine examination. CT scanning is simple, and the scanning speed is fast. It is easy to be clinically performed. It can not only diagnose these four deformities but also accurately diagnose the accompanying extra-cardiac malformation. It clearly shows the development and variation of pulmonary artery and coronary artery, and chooses the surgical method. And the development of surgical plans is of great significance.

20.4　Key Points

- TOF is a cyanotic congenital heart disorder that encompasses four anatomic abnormalities: overriding aorta, ventricular septal defect (VSD), right ventricular hypertrophy, and right ventricular (RV) outflow obstruction.
- The diagnosis of TOF is typically made by MDCT figuring the location and number of

VSDs, the anatomy and severity of RV outflow tract obstruction, the coronary artery and aortic arch anatomy, the presence of any associated anomalies.

References

1. Al Habib HF, Jacobs JP, Mavroudis C, et al. Contemporary patterns of management of tetralogy of Fallot: data from the Society of Thoracic Surgeons Database. Ann Thorac Surg. 2010;90(3):813–9.
2. Centers for Disease Control and Prevention (CDC). Improved national prevalence estimates for 18 selected major birth defects--United States, 1999-2001. MMWR Morb Mortal Wkly Rep. 2006;54(51):1301.
3. Reller MD, Strickland MJ, Riehle-Colarusso T, et al. Prevalence of congenital heart defects in metropolitan Atlanta, 1998-2005. J Pediatr. 2008;153(6):807–13.

Cardiac Myxoma

21

Qian Chen, Song Luo, and Longjiang Zhang

Abstract

Cardiac myxoma (CM) is the commonest primary cardiac tumor. It originates from any chamber of the heart, but mostly occur in the left atrial septum. A CM could induce relative mitral stenosis or regurgitation and even lead to severe hemodynamic abnormalities with the risk of postural syncope, embolism, and sudden death. CM is a benign heart tumor that can be cured by surgical resection. Accurately evaluating tumor initial localization, size, and mobility before surgery, and monitoring the response to surgical outcomes are important for CM's treatment. Cardiac CT can provide guidance for comprehensive clinical evaluation and surgical treatment. In addition, it can clearly depict and evaluate the severity of valvular disease and measure the hemodynamic parameters, which could be used as a favorable supplement to ultrasound. In this chapter, based on a case of CM, we will discuss the cardiac CT imaging manifestations of CM, and further possibly promising role of new cardiac CT technology in CM.

21.1 Case of CM

21.1.1 History

- A 53-year-old male patient had progressive exertional chest tightness for 1 month.
- Transthoracic echocardiography demonstrated a mass in the left atrium in other hospitals.
- He was admitted to our hospital for suspected cardiac tumor.

Physical Examination
- Blood pressure: 120/85 mmHg; Breathing rate: 16/min
- Heart rate: 95 bpm without arrhythmia

Laboratory
- Serum myocardial enzyme spectrum showed negative results.

21.1.2 Imaging Examination

Transthoracic Echocardiography (Fig. 21.1)

Chest Plain X-ray (Fig. 21.2)

CT Images
A coronary CT angiography (CTA) was performed to investigate the coronary artery status and the tumor in the left atrium (Figs. 21.3 and 21.4).

Q. Chen · S. Luo · L. Zhang (✉)
Department of Medical Imaging, Jinling Hospital,
Medical School of Nanjing University,
Nanjing, Jiangsu, China

© Springer Nature Singapore Pte Ltd. 2020
Z.-y. Jin et al. (eds.), *Cardiac CT*, https://doi.org/10.1007/978-981-15-5305-9_21

Fig. 21.1 Transthoracic echocardiography shows a mobile echoic mass in the left atrium attached to the atrial septum

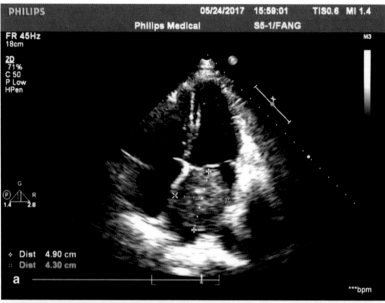

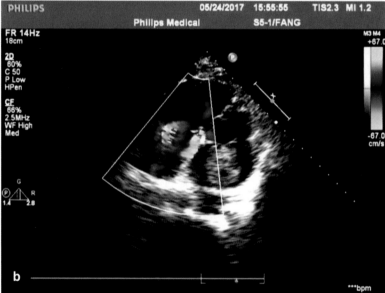

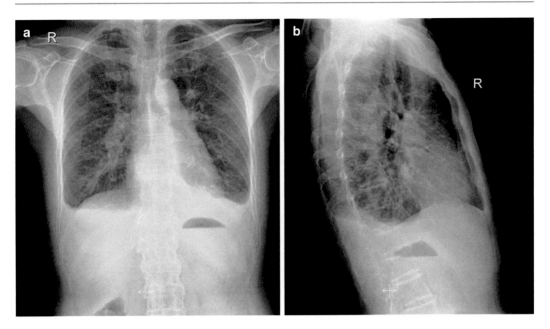

Fig. 21.2 Frontal (**a**) and lateral (**b**) chest plain films show enlarged left atrium and bilateral pleural effusions

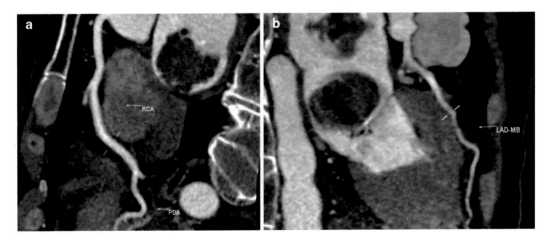

Fig. 21.3 Curved multi-planar (CPR) reconstructed images (**a**, right coronary artery [RCA]; **b**, left anterior descending [LAD] branch) show myocardial bridge in the middle segment of LAD. A low-density mass is shown in the left atrium

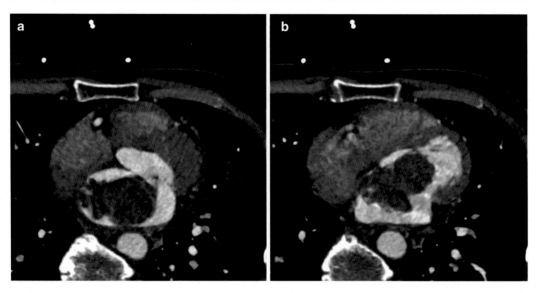

Fig. 21.4 The shape and location of CM in different cardiac cycles. CTA images in the systolic phase (**a**) and in the diastolic phase (**b**) show a dancing, ovoid, and homogeneous mass going back and forth between the left atrium and left ventricle

21.1.3 Imaging Findings and Diagnosis

Transthoracic echocardiography demonstrated a mobile echoic mass in the left atrium attached to the atrial septum. Chest Plain films discovered enlarged left atrium and bilateral pleural effusion. The coronary CTA reconstructed images showed myocardial bridge in the middle segment of LAD. A low-density mass was detected in the left atrium. The different cardiac cycles on CTA images disclosed a dancing, ovoid, and homogeneous mass going back and forth between the left atrium and left ventricle. The patient underwent a cardiac operation and the pathological findings showed the resected tumor was CM.

21.1.4 Management

- The mass was removed by operation.
- Pathological examination showed cardiac myxoma (Fig. 21.5).

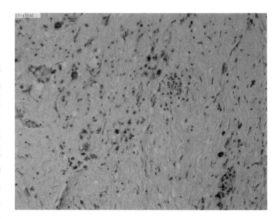

Fig. 21.5 Pathological examination of the mass reveals abundant loose myxoid stroma with myxoma cells (HE staining, ×200)

21.2 Discussion

CM is the most common primary cardiac tumor, comprising up to 50% of the total [1]. Although it can originate from any chamber of the heart, the most majority of CM occur in the left atrial septum.

The endocardial attachment point is either broad, pedunculated, or sessile [2]. The latter are typically mobile and the degree of mobility depends on the length of the stalk. These types of CM may prolapse across the atrioventricular valve during the diastole, thus restricting ventricular filling.

CM is reported to have a mean size of 3–4 cm, while tumor size can be highly variable. The tumor size of CM determines its mobility and its potential for obstructing the atrioventricular valve [3]. Tumor boundaries are either lobulated (most common), smooth, or irregular, with villous expansion or even fragmented appearance. Although CM is considered a benign tumor with a variable vascularization and growth rate, some studies demonstrate its high growth rates mimicking malignant processes [4]. Rarely, atypical CM may be misdiagnosed as malignant tumor such as sarcoma, which shows the presence of mitoses or pleomorphic cells at histology.

Clinical features of CM are variable. Approximately 20% of patients are asymptomatic. Some patients presented with constitutional symptoms, including fever of unknown origin or weight loss. However, CM could also lead to severe hemodynamic abnormalities with the risk of postural syncope, embolism, and sudden death [5].

21.3 Current Technical Status and Applications of CT

During the past decade, several imaging modalities, such as coronary angiography (CA), echocardiography, and cardiac magnetic resonance imaging have been utilized for the study of tumor [6]. Although echocardiography is currently the first line for CMs evaluation, it has several limitations on tumor detection. It is not specific, and is difficult to discriminate other cardiac masses, such as thrombi. CA lacks sensitivity and specificity to distinguish myxoma from thrombi; therefore, it is only suitable for selected patients. Cardiac MRI has some advantages in the evaluation of CMs, due to superior temporal resolution,

soft tissue characterization, and typical signal intensity. However, it has limitations including longer scanning time, higher cost, and MRI cannot be applied in patients with implanted metallic devices [7].

CT is a valuable noninvasive imaging modality that has been used for the evaluation of normal cardiac anatomical structures and adjacent structures. CT images can be reconstructed by multi-planar reconstruction, maximum intensity projection, and volume render (VR) [8]. With these techniques, CT is able to capture fine images of cardiac masses. Therefore, it can be used to depict the morphology character of CMs, and measure the tumor pedicle diameter and originating over time.

In clinical practice, it is important to differentiate cardiac tumors from cardiac tumor-like lesions, such as thrombi, because of the different management of these lesions [9]. CMs and thrombi are usually detected by CT images according to anatomic appearance. As both CMs and thrombi can be localized at the left atrial septum and irregular in shape, it may be challenging to differentiate the two diseases. Several studies have demonstrated that CMs and thrombi are difficult to differentiate based on CT attenuation values [10, 11]. Dual-energy CT is a technological development in imaging, allowing radiologists to differentiate contrast-enhanced structures from otherwise dense high-attenuation materials by using two different X-ray spectra. Recently, dual-energy CT imaging has shown great promise to differentiate between CMs and thrombi [12].

21.4 Key Points

- CM is the most common primary cardiac tumor. It mostly occurs in the left atrium. CM is a benign heart tumor that can be cured by surgical resection.
- CT is an important noninvasive imaging tool to evaluate normal anatomy, including cardiac structures and adjacent anatomical structures.

References

1. Burke AP, Virmani R. Cardiac myxoma. A clinicopathologic study. Am J Clin Pathol. 1993;100(6):671–80.
2. Kosmider A, Jaszewski R, Marcinkiewicz A, et al. 23-year experience on diagnosis and surgical treatment of benign and malignant cardiac tumors. Arch Med Sci. 2013;9(5):826–30.
3. Wei K, Guo HW, Fan SY, et al. Clinical features and surgical results of cardiac myxoma in Carney complex. J Card Surg. 2019;34(1):14–9.
4. Remadi JP, Abdallah L, Tribouilloy C. Huge cardiac myxoma. Ann Thorac Surg. 2017;103(4): e373.
5. Karabinis A, Samanidis G, Khoury M, et al. Clinical presentation and treatment of cardiac myxoma in 153 patients. Medicine (Baltimore). 2018;97(37): e12397.
6. Colin GC, Gerber BL, Amzulescu M, et al. Cardiac myxoma: a contemporary multimodality imaging review. Int J Cardiovasc Imaging. 2018;34(11):1789–808.
7. Kassi M, Polsani V, Schutt RC, et al. Differentiating benign from malignant cardiac tumors with cardiac magnetic resonance imaging. J Thorac Cardiovasc Surg. 2019;157(5):1912–1922.e2.
8. Al JO, Abu SW, Patel AP, et al. Use of three-dimensional models to assist in the resection of malignant cardiac tumors. J Card Surg. 2016;31(9):581–3.
9. Abu AM, Saleh S, Alhaddad E, et al. Cardiac myxoma: clinical characteristics, surgical intervention, intra-operative challenges and outcome. Perfusion. 2017;32(8):686–90.
10. Hans S, Stephan B, Paul S, et al. Atrial myxomas and thrombi: comparison of imaging features on CT. AJR Am J Roentgenol. 2009;192(3):639–45.
11. Claussen C, Hler DK, Schartl M, et al. Computer tomographic and echocardiographic diagnosis of intracardial space occupying masses. Rofo. 1983;138(3):296–301.
12. Hong YJ, Hur J, Kim YJ, et al. Dual-energy cardiac computed tomography for differentiating cardiac myxoma from thrombus. Int J Cardiovasc Imaging. 2014;30(Suppl 2):121–8.

Fibroma

22

Fan Yang, Zhang Zhang, and Dong Li

Abstract

Fibroma is a benign tumor that occurs most commonly in children and may be associated with Gorlin syndrome. It is predominantly detected in the left ventricle. Accurate diagnosis is crucial for the perioperative management of these patients. Generally, echocardiography was the first-line examination for screening abnormality including cardiac mass. Cardiac magnetic resonance imaging was the multiparameter method for the evaluation of fibroma. Cardiac computed tomography (CT) (both pre-contrast and post-contrast) could be used for evaluation and diagnosis of tumor as well, which include assessing the location and extent of mass, whether the surrounding structure of the heart is invasive, and the possible tissue composition. In this chapter, we will show cardiac CT imaging manifestations of fibroma.

22.1 Case of Fibroma

22.1.1 History

- An 82-year-old female patient felt discomfort on intermittent upper abdomen.

Physical Examination
- Blood pressure: 156/84 mmHg; Breathing rate: 25/min
- Heart rate: 86 bpm without arrhythmia

Electrocardiograph
- Standard 12-lead electrocardiograph (ECG) revealed ST-T segment changes on leads V4–V6 and T wave inversion.

Laboratory
- Serum myocardial enzyme spectrum and NTpro-BNP results were within the reference ransge.

22.1.2 Imaging Examination

CT Images
Coronary CT angiography (CTA) was requested to investigate the coronary artery status and other potential cardiomyopathies (Figs. 22.1, 22.2, 22.3, and 22.4).

F. Yang · Z. Zhang · D. Li (✉)
Radiology Department, Tianjin Medical University
General Hospital, Tianjin, China

© Springer Nature Singapore Pte Ltd. 2020
Z.-y. Jin et al. (eds.), *Cardiac CT*, https://doi.org/10.1007/978-981-15-5305-9_22

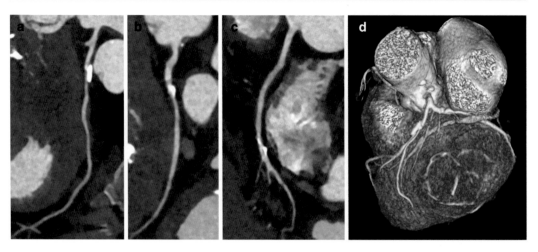

Fig. 22.1 Curved multi-planar reformat (CPR) images (**a**, left anterior descending [LAD] branch; **b**, left circumflex artery [LCX]); **c**, right coronary artery [RCA]) and volume rendering (VR) image (**d**) of the coronary CTA. Calcified plaques were detected in three coronary arteries with moderate stenosis. VR image showed multiple stripe-like high-density opacities in the lateral wall of the left ventricle (LV)

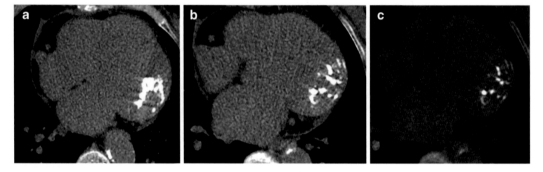

Fig. 22.2 Non-contrast CT axial view images (**a**–**c**) showed thickened myocardium of LV lateral wall with multiple nodular, stripe-like, and irregular calcifications

22.1.3 Imaging Findings and Diagnosis

The coronary CTA images results showed that there were calcified plaques in the proximal segments of LAD and LCX and middle-distal segment of RCA, resulted in moderate lumen stenosis. All the cardiac view of multi-planar reformats, including short-axial view, four-chamber view, and two-chamber view, showed the asymmetric myocardial hypertrophy and a well-defined mass within the lateral wall of LV. The mass was of relatively low density to myocardium and showed dissipate nodular, stripe-like, and irregular calcifications inside the mass. In addition, pericardial effusion was minimal.

22.1.4 Management

- Complete resection therapy for the mass
- Out-patient follow-up observations for cardiac function and recurrence of the tumor

22.2 Discussion

Fibroma is a hamartomatous benign lesion that is present from birth with a mean age of onset at 11 years and rarely detected in adults [1]. The ventricle is the frequent site of involvement. The tumor cells resemble fibroblasts with variable collagen and elastic tissue and commonly contain calcifications. Cardiac fibromas are

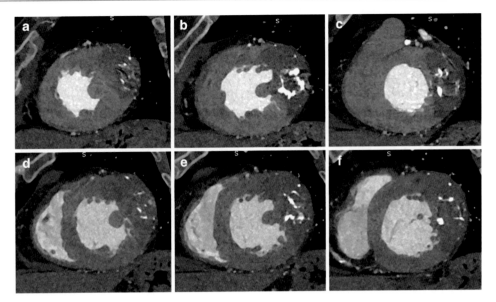

Fig. 22.3 Cardiac CT imaging of myocardium in short-axial view in systolic phase (**a–c**) and diastolic phase (**e–f**) showed asymmetric thickened myocardium in LV and septum and an ovate mass in the lateral wall of LV, pre-senting as relative low density to myocardium and multi-ple calcifications, without obvious enhancement. The pericardium showed mild pericardial effusion

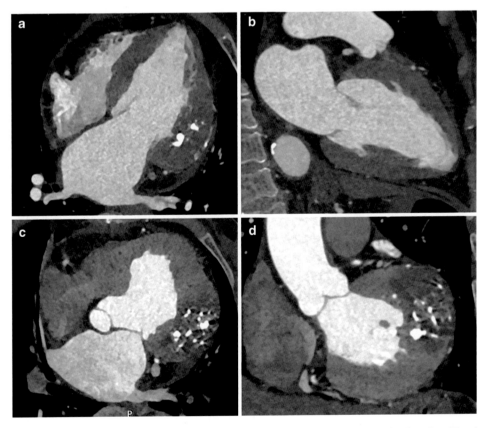

Fig. 22.4 Cardiac CT imaging of myocardium in four-chamber (**a, c**) view, long-axial two-chamber view (**b**) and coro-nal view (**d**) exhibited myocardial hypertrophy and the relative well-defined mass

associated with an autosomal dominant disease called Gorlin syndrome (also known as nevoid basal cell carcinoma syndrome) that is characterized by skin cancer, unusual brain tumors, skeletal abnormalities, and macrocephaly [1]. Patients may have unspecific signs and symptoms including ventricular arrhythmias, cyanosis, dyspnea, and sudden death. Up to one-third of the patients can be asymptomatic even until their old age. Patients may have electrocardiographic findings similar to those with hypertrophic myocardiopathy (HCM). Mass in the LV with calcification is the characteristic imaging finding on CT. Compensated myocardial hypertrophy can be seen. Cardiac CT is sensitive for differential diagnosis with HCM. Tumors in symptomatic patients should be treated by complete resection and postoperative prognosis is typically well. Some patients may require heart transplantation [2].

22.3   Current Technical Status and Applications of CT

On cardiac CT imaging, fibromas manifest as well-defined, solitary, intramural, homogenous masses with soft-tissue attenuation in noncontrast enhanced scan. The infiltrative profile is not uncommon. Fibroma usually does not perform cyst, focal necrosis, or hemorrhage, whereas calcification is common. They are commonly located in the left ventricular free wall and ventricular septum and rarely in the atrium [2]. The location and morphology of the mass is crucial for treatment decision.

After contrast injection, fibromas are usually hypoattenuating relative to the myocardium in the arterial and venous (early and late) phases and homogeneously as progressively slightly enhanced. These neoplasms are avascular and thus do not usually exhibit enhancement during perfusion imaging [3]. Characteristically, fibromas are obviously enhancement on late gadolinium enhancement (LGE) MR imaging applicated in the 8–15 min later after contrast injection.

Cardiac CT examination could reveal a lot for diagnosis and treatment choice and pre-operation preparation.

22.4   Key Points

- Cardiac fibroma is a rare benign tumor predominantly occurring in LV. Patients with fibroma may have electrocardiographic findings similar to those with HCM.
- Cardiac CT examination with reconstruction technology may be helpful to correct differential diagnosis of fibroma from HCM and delineate the mass and internal characteristics.

References

1. Burke A, Tavora F. The 2015 WHO classification of tumors of the heart and pericardium. J Thorac Oncol. 2016;11(4):441–52.
2. Maleszewski JJ, Anavekar NS, Moynihan TJ, Klarich KW. Pathology, imaging, and treatment of cardiac tumours. Nat Rev Cardiol. 2017;14(9):536–49.
3. Lichtenberger JP, Dulberger AR, Gonzales PE, et al. MR imaging of cardiac masses. Top Magn Reson Imaging. 2018;27(2):103–11.

Mesothelioma

23

Fan Yang, Zhang Zhang, and Dong Li

Abstract

Mesothelioma is a rare tumor that mostly exhibits massive tumors with or without pericardium effusion, even associated with myocardial infiltration. Massive effusion and diffused irregular thickening of the pericardium may lead to tamponade and constriction. Clinically, no definite relationship between pericardial mesothelioma and asbestos exposure has been identified. Diffused spreading throughout on the pericardium leads to poor prognosis. Though mesothelioma is extremely rare, we should identify the tumor and make differential diagnosis. In this chapter, we will discuss the cardiac computed tomography (CT) imaging manifestations of mesothelioma.

23.1 Case of Mesothelioma

23.1.1 History

- A 61-year-old female patient presents with chest pain and night sweats for 4 months.
- He had a recent fever for more than 2 weeks.

F. Yang · Z. Zhang · D. Li (✉)
Radiology Department, Tianjin Medical University General Hospital, Tianjin, China

- Echocardiography indicated that a mass was found in front of ascending aorta and right ventricle (RV).

Physical Examination

- Blood pressure: 150/95 mmHg; Breathing rate: 24/min.
- Heart rate: 107 bpm without arrhythmia; no murmur was detected.

Laboratory

Serum tumor markers results showed that carbohydrate antigen125 (CA125) (636.0 U/ml) and tissue polypeptide specific antigen (TPS) (138.46 U/L) were elevated.

23.1.2 Imaging Examination

CT Images

Coronary CT angiography (CTA) combined with calcium scoring images was requested to investigate the coronary artery status and delineate the mass (Figs. 23.1, 23.2, 23.3, and 23.4).

23.1.3 Imaging Findings and Diagnosis

The coronary CTA images results showed no plaque, stenosis, and dilation has been found in all the coronary arteries. Primary and recon-

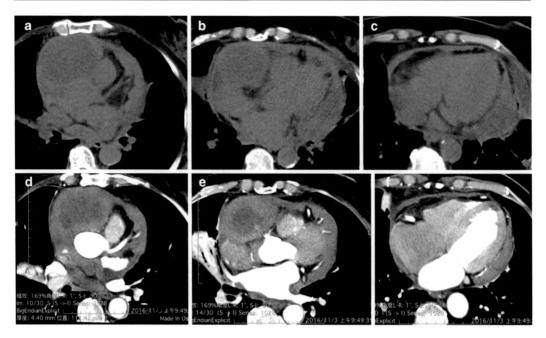

Fig. 23.1 Calcium scoring (non-contrast enhancement) images (**a–c**) and axial cardiac images (**d–f**) of the coronary CTA showed diffused irregular thickening of the pericardium with slight enhancement and a mass in front of the right atrium (RA) and RV. The mass manifested heterogeneous enhancement with central necrosis. Subcarinal lymphadenectasis and infiltrated fat tissue were detected

structed images showed diffused irregular thickening of the pericardium with slight enhancement and a mass in front of RA and RV surrounding the ascending aorta and main pulmonary artery. The mass manifested apparent heterogeneous enhancement with central necrosis. Mediastinal lymphadenectasis was detected in the subcarinal space. The irregular thickened pericardium had infiltrated the fat tissue in the mediastinum. One-year later, after diagnosis by pericardiocentesis, the lesions in the pericardium had aggressive progression.

23.1.4 Management

- Radiotherapy or chemotherapy for unresectable masses
- Close follow-up by CT for recurrent and metastasis

23.2 Discussion

Primary pericardial mesothelioma is rare, though it is the most common primary pericardial malignancy [1]. Most of the mesotheliomas are malignant. There is a 2:1 male–female ratio and over half of the cases occur in the fifth through seventh decades of life [2]. Massive tumors with or without pericardium effusion may lead to tamponade and constriction, and myocardial infiltration which may result in conduction abnormalities. Invasion of the underlying myocardium is not uncommon. Unlike pleural mesothelioma, no definite relationship between pericardial mesothelioma and asbestos exposure has been identified. Effusion commonly shows hemorrhagic fluid with cytology revealed malignant cells in only 20% of cases [3].

Although resection is the treatment of choice for mesothelioma, most of the tumors are unable

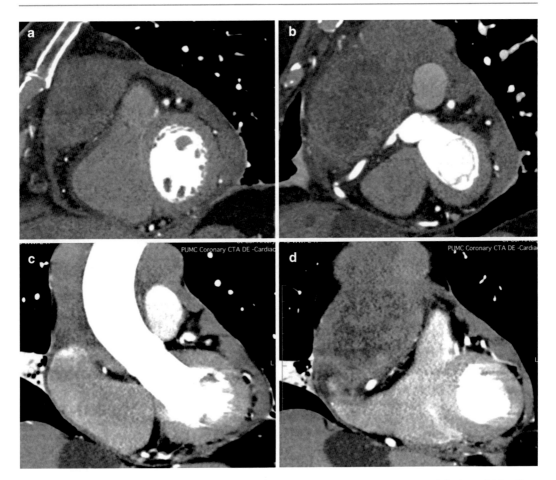

Fig. 23.2 Short axial cardiac images (**a, b**) and coronal reconstruction CT images (**c, d**) showed diffused irregular thickening of pericardium surrounding the ascending aorta, main pulmonary artery, and the heart. Epicardium of the left ventricle could not be separated from the thickened pericardium

to completely eradicate it surgically because of diffused spreading throughout on the pericardium [2]. Furthermore, response to radiotherapy or chemotherapy is poor.

Clinically, differential diagnosis is of great importance in patients with multiple nodules in the pericardium because lymphoma, metastasis, and granulomatosis could have a similar manifestation.

23.3 Current Technical Status and Applications of CT

The sensitivity of echocardiography in the detection of pericardial mesothelioma is low.

Fortunately, CT offers an advantage result from better depict the extent of involvement of contiguous structures and the degree of constriction. Pericardial mesothelioma typically appears as diffused irregular pericardial thickening or multiple nodules that involves both the parietal and visceral layers of the pericardium associated with pericardial effusion. The tumors are commonly heterogeneously enhancing. Most of the lesions are invasive and may invade the adjacent vascular and anatomic structures around pericardium. CT can detect metastasis which could be found in approximately 50% of the cases, most commonly in local mediastinal lymph nodes and the lungs.

Appropriate cardiac CT examination contributes a lot for correct differential diagnosis think-

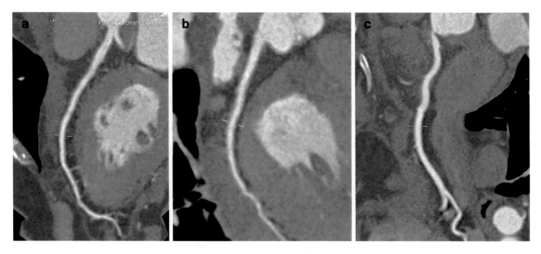

Fig. 23.3 Curved multi-planar reformats (CPR) images (**a**, left anterior descending [LAD] branch; **b**, left circumflex artery [LCX]; **c**, right coronary artery) of the coronary CTA showed no plaque, stenosis, and dilation on the coronary arteries

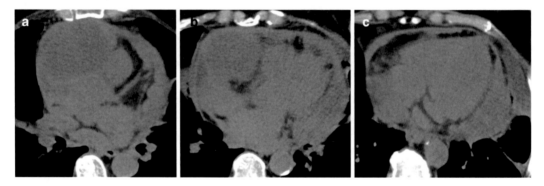

Fig. 23.4 One year after diagnosis by pericardiocentesis non-contrast enhanced axial CT images showed the progressive thickening of pericardial masses

ing and prompt treatment choice, as well as accurate prognosis assessment.

23.4   Key Points

- Mesothelioma is often aggressive and could infiltrate the adjacent tissue and structure, even the myocardium.
- CT imaging including with and without contrast enhancement was capable of detecting and evaluating the scope and infiltration of lesion, which is helpful to diagnosis and follow-up.

References

1. Zhou W, Srichai MB. Multi-modality imaging assessment of pericardial masses. Curr Cardiol Rep. 2017;19(4):32.
2. Restrepo CS, Vargas D, Ocazionez D, et al. Primary pericardial tumors. Radiographics. 2013;33(6):1613–30.
3. Lamba G, Frishman WH. Cardiac and pericardial tumors. Cardiol Rev. 2012;20(5):237–52.

Cardiac Sarcoma

24

Qian Chen, Song Luo, and Longjiang Zhang

Abstract

Primary cardiac neoplasms are extremely rare. The majority of tumors are benign (75%). Of the remaining 25% of tumors that are identified as being malignant, cardiac sarcomas comprise 95% of cases. Primary cardiac angiosarcoma is the most common histological subtype and constitutes 30% of those cases. Echocardiography is the screening modality of choice. MRI and CT are complementary to echocardiography in aiding the diagnosis of cardiac malignancy. Cardiac CT allows the evaluation of the tumor burden and vascularity to help distinguish this rare malignant tumor. In this chapter, based on a case of cardiac angiosarcoma, we will discuss the cardiac CT imaging manifestations of sarcoma.

24.1 Case of Cardiac Angiosarcoma

24.1.1 History

- A 59-year-old female patient had no obvious cause of facial edema for 1 month and felt repeated chest tightness for 2 weeks.

- Transthoracic echocardiography revealed massive pericardial effusion in another hospital.
- She was sent to perform cardiac CT for suspected cardiac disease.

Physical Examination
- Blood pressure: 122/74 mmHg
- Breathing rate: 18/min
- Heart rate: 92 bpm

Electrocardiograph
Standard 12-lead electrocardiograph (ECG) revealed paroxysmal atrial fibrillation.

Laboratory
Blood routine and blood biochemical parameters showed severe degree of anemia and hypoproteinemia.

24.1.2 Imaging Examination

^{18}F-FDG PET-CT Images
The patient received a PET-CT scan to detect malignant tumors (Fig. 24.1).

CT Images
A cardiac CT scan was performed to investigate the cardiac structure and coronary artery status (Figs. 24.2 and 24.3).

Q. Chen · S. Luo · L. Zhang (✉)
Department of Medical Imaging, Jinling Hospital,
Medical School of Nanjing University,
Nanjing, Jiangsu, China

© Springer Nature Singapore Pte Ltd. 2020
Z.-y. Jin et al. (eds.), *Cardiac CT*, https://doi.org/10.1007/978-981-15-5305-9_24

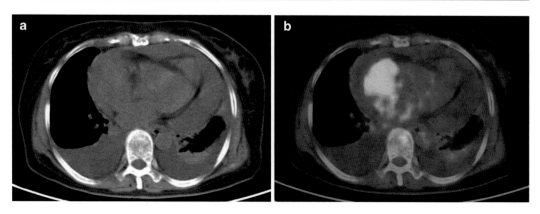

Fig. 24.1 ¹⁸F-FDG PET-CT (**a**, **b**) reveal a soft tissue mass with increased ¹⁸F-FDG uptake in the right atrium

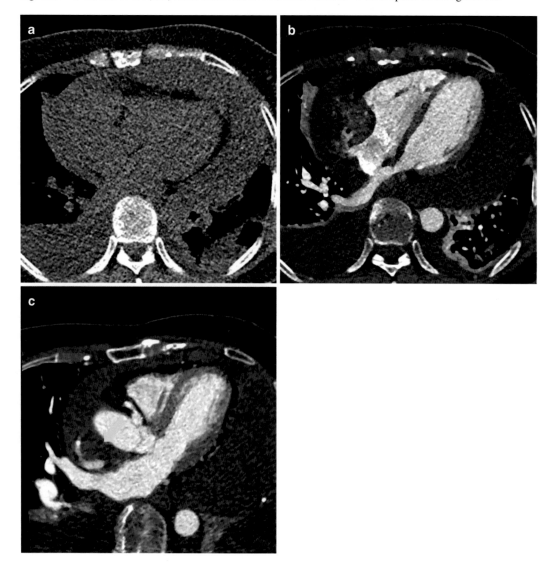

Fig. 24.2 Plain cardiac CT image (**a**) shows massive pericardial effusion and bilateral pleural effusion. Contrast-enhanced cardiac CT images (**b**, **c**) demonstrate an oval, well-defined mass with heterogeneous enhance-

ment centered in the right atrium. The mass involved the right atrial wall and extended outside the right atrium, partly enclosed the superior vena cava, which was compressed to become flat (arrow)

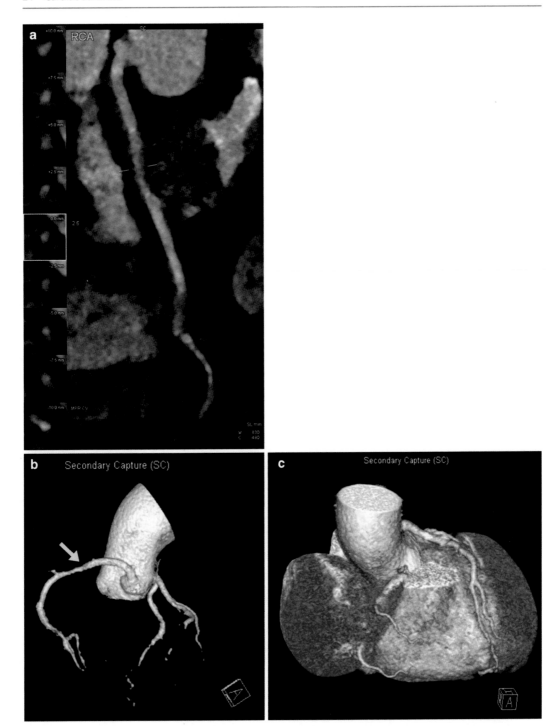

Fig. 24.3 Curved multi-planar (CPR) reconstructed image (**a**, right coronary artery [RCA]), and volume render (VR) images (**b**, **c**) show the mass involved the middle segment of RCA, which shows mild stenosis

24.1.3 Imaging Findings and Diagnosis

The cardiac CT showed an oval, round margin mass with heterogeneous enhancement centered in the right atrium. The mass involved the right atrial wall and extended outside the right atrium. The proximal-middle segment of RCA was surrounded by the mass and demonstrated mild stenosis. The superior vena cava was partially enclosed and compressed to become flat. Massive pericardial effusion and bilateral pleural effusion were discovered. A malignant cardiac tumor was considered according to the imaging features.

24.1.4 Management

* The mass was partially removed by operation.
* Pathological examination showed cardiac angiosarcoma (Fig. 24.4).
* Recurrence was found in the 3 months follow-up CT examination (Fig. 24.5).

24.2 Discussion

Primary cardiac tumors are rare with an incidence between 0.0017% and 0.019% [1]. Twenty-five percent of cardiac tumors are malignant [2]. Primary malignant cardiac tumors are predominantly sarcomas in nature. Angiosarcoma

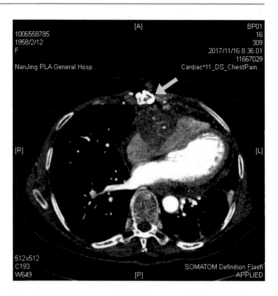

Fig. 24.5 Three months follow-up CT image shows recurrence of the tumor. Note the metal suture in the sternal (arrow)

is the most prevalent primary cardiac malignant tumor, which is mostly originated from the right atrial free wall [3, 4]. The typical morphology of angiosarcoma consists of a large, multi-lobulated mass with a heterogeneous composition that extends along the epicardial surface and replaces the right atrial wall. Given the bulky nature, it may involve the right coronary artery leading to rupture [5]. Angiosarcoma may also be originated from the pericardium and often involves adjacent cardiac structures resulting in cardiomegaly and recurrent pericardial effusions [6].

Clinical symptoms usually present with right-sided heart failure or cardiac tamponade. Other presenting symptoms include hemoptysis secondary to diffuse pulmonary hemorrhage and clinical features related to metastasis. The clinical course of angiosarcoma is rapid and the prognosis is usually poor, due to the difficulties in surgery, with a high rate of local recurrence and metastases [7].

24.3 Current Technical Status and Applications of CT

Transthoracic echocardiography remains the first-line diagnostic modality to assess cardiac masses. The advantages of echocardiography

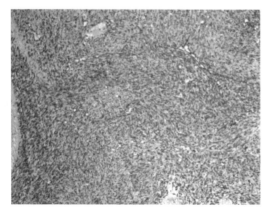

Fig. 24.4 Pathological examination of the mass demonstrates abundant spindle cells of cardiac angiosarcoma (HE staining, ×100)

include no radiation or contrast exposure, widespread availability, and real-time assessment of cardiac activity. Major limitations include operator dependence, inability to determine the full extent and origin of a mass due to restricted field-of-view, and little capacity for tissue characterization [8]. Cardiac MR has been shown to be the preferred imaging test for the detection of cardiac masses, and is recommended for pediatric patients, where radiation is a concern [9]. Cardiac CT is an excellent tool for the evaluation of calcified masses and concurrent coronary artery invasion, which may impact the operation time and decision-making.

Cardiac CT allows assessment of the tumor morphology, size, and vascularity to help distinguish the rare malignant tumor. There are two main morphologic types of angiosarcoma [10]. The first is a well-defined mass protruding into a cardiac chamber, usually the right atrium. The atrial septum is often spared. At gross examination, the tumors are necrotic, hemorrhagic, and usually adhere to the pericardium. CT often reveals a low attenuation right atrial mass, which may be nodular or irregular and usually originates from the right atrial free wall. Central areas of necrosis in communication with a cardiac chamber have been described at CT. CT can demonstrate tumor infiltration through the myocardium, compression of cardiac chambers, involvement of the great vessels, and direct extension into the pericardium [11]. The tumor can have heterogeneous contrast enhancement on contrast-enhanced CT. The second morphologic type is a diffusely infiltrative mass extending along the pericardium. The pericardial space may be obliterated with necrotic tumor debris and hemorrhage, which may appear as pericardial thickening or effusion on CT [12].

24.4   Key Points

- Cardiac angiosarcoma is the most prevalent primary cardiac malignant tumor. The tumors tend to occur in the right atrium and involve the pericardium.

- Cardiac CT examination allows the evaluation of the tumor and adjacent structures including the myocardium, pericardium, mediastinum, great vessels, and pulmonary metastasis.

References

1. Silverman NA. Primary cardiac tumors. Ann Surg. 1980;191(2):127–38.
2. Hudzik B, Miszalski-Jamka K, Glowacki J, et al. Malignant tumors of the heart. Cancer Epidemiol. 2015;39(5):665–72.
3. Butany J, Nair V, Naseemuddin A, et al. Cardiac tumours: diagnosis and management. Lancet Oncol. 2005;6(4):219–28.
4. Tacket HS, Jones RS, Kyle JW. Primary angiosarcoma of the heart. Am Heart J. 1950;39(6):912–7.
5. Tang K, Shang QL, Zhou QC, et al. Primary cardiac angiosarcoma with spontaneous ruptures of the right atrium and right coronary artery. Echocardiography. 2014;30(6):E156–60.
6. Eric R, Suraj G, Dee Dee W, et al. Primary cardiac angiosarcoma: a diagnostic challenge in a young man with recurrent pericardial effusions. Exp Clin Cardiol. 2012;17(1):39–42.
7. Dichek DA, Holmvang G, Fallon JT, et al. Angiosarcoma of the heart: Three-year survival and follow-up by nuclear magnetic resonance imaging. Am Heart J. 1988;115(6):1323–4.
8. Valecha G, Pau D, Nalluri N, et al. Primary intimal sarcoma of the left atrium: an incidental finding on routine echocardiography. Rare Tumors. 2016;8(4):6389.
9. Klein AL, Abbara S, Agler DA, et al. American Society of Echocardiography clinical recommendations for multimodality cardiovascular imaging of patients with pericardial disease: endorsed by the society for cardiovascular magnetic resonance and Society of Cardiovascular Computed Tomography. J Am Soc Echocardiogr. 2013;26(9):965–1012.e15.
10. El-Osta HE, Yammine YS, Chehab BM, et al. Unexplained hemopericardium as a presenting feature of primary cardiac angiosarcoma: a case report and a review of the diagnostic dilemma. J Thorac Oncol. 2008;3(7):800–2.
11. Heenan S, Ignotus P, Cox I, et al. Case report: percutaneous biopsy of a right atrial angiosarcoma under ultrasound guidance. Clin Radiol. 1996;51(8):591–2.
12. Goradia D, Chew FS. Cardiac angiosarcoma on CT. Radiol Case Rep. 2006;1(4):126–7.

Paraganglioma

25

Lu Lin and Yining Wang

Abstract

Primary cardiac paraganglioma is an extremely rare cardiac tumor but with classic clinical and imaging characteristics. The diagnosis can be made on the basis of clinical manifestation (hypertension and evidence of catecholamine overproduction), biochemical lab tests, and nuclear medicine imaging most of the time. Contrast-enhanced CT is an essential complementary imaging technology to evaluate the lesion's range, blood supply, and anatomic relation to adjacent structures, which provide useful information to operation planning. Cardiac paraganglioma is commonly iso-attenuating with adjacent cardiovascular structures in non-contrast CT imaging, but evidently enhanced after contrast for its hyper-vascular nature. Feeding arteries from coronary circulation can be delineated clearly by coronary CT angiography. Advances in multi-detector CT hardware and more sophisticated post-processing technique have made 3D reconstructions a useful adjunct in imaging assessment. Three-dimensional printing based on CT is an emerging technology which may offer additional value for the operation.

L. Lin · Y. Wang (✉)
Department of Radiology, Peking Union Medical College Hospital, Chinese Academy of Medical Sciences and Peking Union Medical College, Beijing, China
e-mail: wangyining@pumch.cn

25.1 Case of Cardiac Paraganglioma

25.1.1 History

A 13-year-old male patient has had excessive perspiration after activities for 5 years without seeing a doctor. A month ago, he had blurred vision, so he went to the local hospital. Prominent increased blood pressure and heart rate were found (233/178 mm Hg; 136 beats per minute). After combined administration of multiple anti-hypertensive drugs (α receptor blocker, β receptor blocker, calcium channel blocker, and ARB), his blood pressure (BP) was controlled to 110–130/60–70 mm Hg.

Physical Examination
Postural hypotension, warm limb terminals, and no abnormal heart murmurs were found.

- Supine position: BP: 101/53 mm Hg (right upper limb), 125/80 mm Hg (left upper limb); heart rate: 76 bpm.
- Standing position: BP: 72/30 mm Hg (right upper limb), 99/48 mm Hg (left upper limb); heart rate: 93 bpm.

Electrocardiograph
Standard 12-lead electrocardiograph (ECG) revealed no obvious abnormality.

© Springer Nature Singapore Pte Ltd. 2020
Z.-y. Jin et al. (eds.), *Cardiac CT*, https://doi.org/10.1007/978-981-15-5305-9_25

Laboratory

- Elevated serum Norepinephrine (NE): 25.4 ng/ml (0.2–0.38).
- Elevated 24 h urinary catecholamine (UCA): NE 1181.32 μg (16.69–40.65), epinephrine (E) 6.76 μg (1.74–6.42), dopamine (DA) 1692.52 μg (120.93–330.59).
- Serum myocardial enzyme spectrum showed negative results.

25.1.2 Imaging Examination

Echocardiography

- A mixed medium echoic mass was found between aortic root, main pulmonary artery, and right chamber outflow, the size of which was about 65 mm × 47 mm. The lesion was ill-defined with unclear demarcation between the great arteries.
- Mild left ventricle hypertrophy with no cardia chambers enlargement.
- Left ventricular ejection fraction (LVEF): 75%.

CT Images

An ECG-triggered cardiac CT angiography was performed to show the mass and its relationship with great and coronary arteries.

- Non-contrast images showed a large low-density mass (average CT value: 30HU) in medium mediastinum, with unclear demarcation between the great arteries (Fig. 25.1a).
- In arterial phase-enhanced images, the mass showed obvious inhomogeneous enhancement (average CT value 120HU) and abundant blood supply, with compression changes of peripheral great vessels and coronary arteries (Fig. 25.1b–d).
- Coronary arteries reconstructed images showed multiple supplying vessels from both left and right coronary arteries (Fig. 25.2).

Nuclear Medicine Imaging

- Somatostatin receptor imaging: a mass near ascending aorta in pericardium showed high expression, which is conformed to paraganglioma (Fig. 25.3).
- Iodine-131 metaiodobenzylguanidine (I-131 MIBG) imaging: high expression mass in mediastinum considered to be paraganglioma.

Conventional Coronary Angiography

X-ray coronary angiography showed widespread tumor stains, enriching blood supply vessels, and

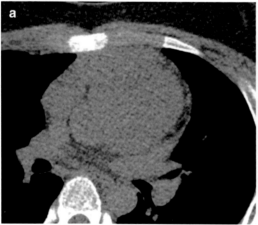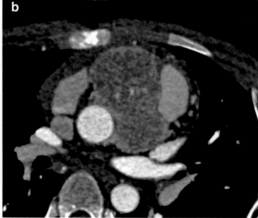

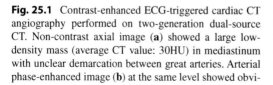

Fig. 25.1 Contrast-enhanced ECG-triggered cardiac CT angiography performed on two-generation dual-source CT. Non-contrast axial image (**a**) showed a large low-density mass (average CT value: 30HU) in mediastinum with unclear demarcation between great arteries. Arterial phase-enhanced image (**b**) at the same level showed obvi-ous inhomogeneous enhancement of the lesion (average CT value 120HU). Coronal reconstructed images (**c–d**) showed abundant supplying vessels of the mass and secondary compression of the main pulmonary artery and left main coronary artery

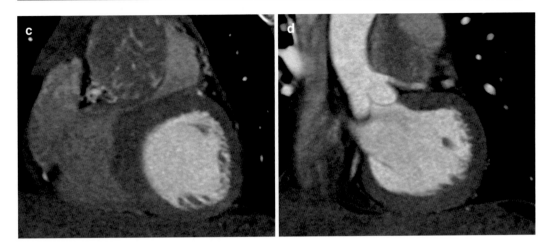

Fig. 25.1 (continued)

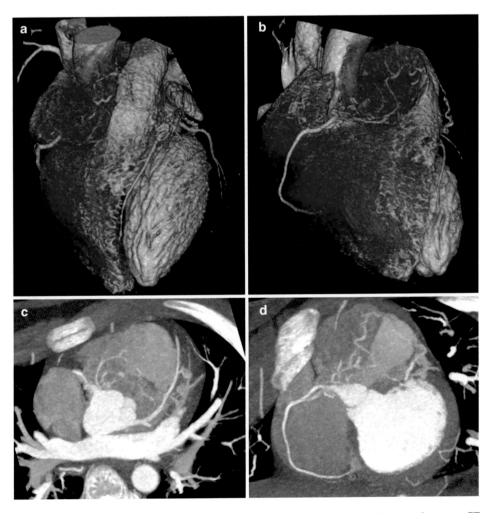

Fig. 25.2 Volume rendering (**a–b**) and maximum intensity projection (**c-d**) reconstructed images of coronary CT angiography. Multiple supplying vessels of the mass were found originated from proximal RCA, proximal and middle LAD

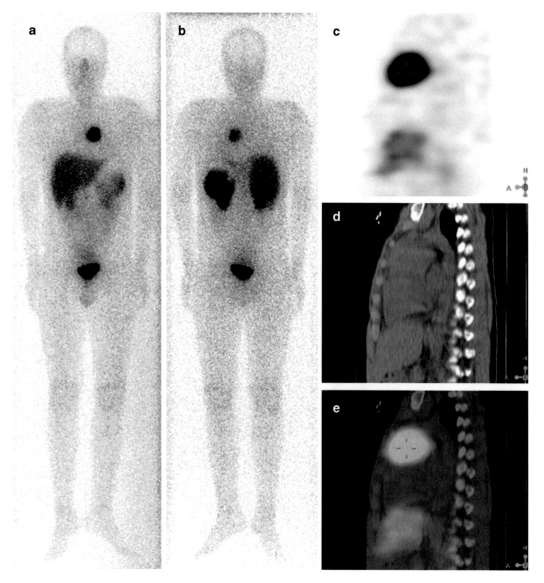

Fig. 25.3 Somatostatin receptor image. Whole-body (**a**-**b**) and sagittal (**c**) radionuclide images displayed a solitary high expression mass in Mediastinum. Fusion image (**e**) with CT (**d**) showed the lesion located in pericardium near the aortic root and main pulmonary artery

collateral circulation. The tumor was mainly supplied by branches from proximal LAD, diagonal and proximal RCA (Fig. 25.4).

25.1.3 Imaging Findings and Diagnosis

The patient is a teenage boy with severe hypertension. Firstly, echocardiography found a large mass between aortic root, main pulmonary artery, and right chamber outflow. Mild left ventricle hypertrophy might be secondary to hypertension. In echo, the lesion was ill-defined and its relationship with peripheral vessels was unclear.

Further ECG-triggered cardiac angiography solved the problem of echo. In CT, the mass was soft tissue density with prominent enhancement and abundant blood supply. Its adjacent great vessels including ascending aortic artery and

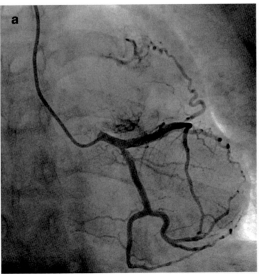
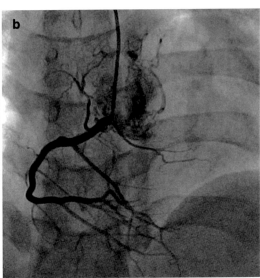

Fig. 25.4 Conventional coronary angiography. X-ray images of left (**a**) and right (**b**) coronary artery displayed three main tumor supplying arteries originated from prox-imal LAD, diagonal and proximal RCA. Widespread tumor stains, enriching blood supply vessels, and collateral circulation were found

main pulmonary artery displayed mainly compression changes instead of being invaded. In coronary CTA reconstructed images, the lesion's supplying vessels were from both left and right coronary arteries and abundant vessels could be seen inside the tumor, which were proved precisely in conventional coronary angiography. The first differential diagnosis should be cardiac paraganglioma. Specific radionuclide imaging and endocrine lab tests supported this diagnosis.

25.1.4 Management

- Strict preoperative drug preparation was given to the patient to control blood pressure and heart rate stability.
- Then he underwent cardiac mass resection, coronary artery bypass grafting (AO-SV-LAD, AO-SV-RCA), right ventricular outflow tract reconstruction and aortic repair under general anesthesia and hypothermic cardiopulmonary bypass.
- Operative findings: The tumor was located between the ascending aorta and the main pulmonary artery, supplied by coronary arteries. The left side of the aortic root and the anterior wall of the right ventricular out-

flow tract were surrounded by a tumor. The main pulmonary artery was compressed and deformed, left main coronary artery invasion was suspected. During operation, the anterior wall of the main pulmonary artery and right ventricular outflow tract were damaged and repaired.

- Postoperative pathology: cardiac paraganglioma; AE1/AE3 (-), CgA (+), Ki-67 (index 3%), Melan-A (-), S-100 (+), A-inhibin (-).
- Post-operation cardiac CT angiography: the bypass vessels were patent and no residual tumor tissue was found.

25.2 Discussion

Primary cardiac neoplasms are rare with a reported prevalence in autopsy series of 0.001–0.03%. It is estimated that primary cardiac neoplasms are 100–1000 times less prevalent than secondary neoplasms [1].

Cardiac paragangliomas arise from intrinsic cardiac paraganglial (chromaffin) cells and are extremely rare, which are predominantly originated from atria. Patients ages range from the early teens to the mid-60s but typically are young adults in their 30s and 40s. Hypertension and bio-chemical evidence of catecholamine overproduc-tion (headache, palpitations, and flushing etc.) are most common presentations. The biochemi-cal laboratory abnormalities include elevated lev-els of urinary norepinephrine, vanillylmandelic acid, and total metanephrine or elevated levels of plasma norepinephrine and epinephrine. Up to 20% of patients with cardiac paragangliomas have paragangliomas in other locations (carotid body, adrenal gland, paraaortic, etc.). Although there are several familial syndromes associated with paragangliomas, nearly all cases of cardiac paraganglioma reported are sporadic [2].

Cardiac paragangliomas are large masses that typically measure 2–14 cm in greatest dimension. The tumors may be encapsulated, but may also be infiltrative. Most lesions are located on the epi-cardial surface of the heart base, in the roof, or posterior wall of the left atrium; less common locations include the atrial cavity, interatrial sep-tum, and ventricles. Most of the tumors are sup-plied by coronary arteries [3].

Radiologic evaluation of paragangliomas usu-ally follows abnormal biochemical exam results. If abdominal imaging studies fail to reveal a typi-cal adrenal pheochromocytoma, nuclear imaging is used to localize the occult lesion. Nuclear imaging is useful for the evaluation of suspected paragangliomas. 123I/131I-MIBG scintigraphy is the initial recommended study but is associated with a high false-negative rate, as the sensitivity is 18–50%. Octreotide scintigraphy and 18F-FDG PET are useful secondary nuclear scans [4].

Echocardiography is the first-line imaging modality for intracardiac disease providing high-resolution, real-time images. At echocardiogra-phy, paragangliomas usually appear as large, echogenic masses. Unlike myxomas, paragangli-omas have a broad attachment base. Compression of adjacent structures such as the superior vena cava may be seen. Encasement of the coronary arteries may be demonstrated [2].

CT demonstrates the morphology, location, and extent of a cardiac neoplasm adequately. Compared with echocardiography, CT has better depiction of pericardium, great vessels, and other extracardiac structures, including metastases.

Coronary angiography optimally reveals the rela-tionship between cardiac mass and coronary arteries including tumor blood supply [5], which is critical for preoperative assessment. Cardiac paragangliomas may be missed on unenhanced chest CT scans because they are commonly iso-attenuating with adjacent structures. However, it should be noted that intravenous contrast mate-rial can trigger a hypertensive crisis in paragan-glioma patients; therefore, premedication with alpha and beta blockers is necessary. Typically, a dynamic contrast-enhanced chest CT reveals a markedly enhancing mass. Approximately half of these lesions have central areas of low attenua-tion, most likely representing necrosis. Tumoral calcification may also be identified. The differen-tial diagnosis of a hyper-enhancing cardiac mass in CT should include angiosarcoma and hyper-vascular metastasis such as melanoma.

MR imaging typically demonstrates a mass that is iso- or hypointense to myocardium on T1-weighted and very hyperintense on T2-weighted images. Increased signal intensity on T1-weighted images is presumably due to hemorrhage in tumor. The intrapericardial loca-tion of the mass and its relationship to the cardio-vascular structures is usually clearly depicted.

The only curative treatment for cardiac paragan-glioma is complete surgical resection. The opera-tion is often complicated by serious hemorrhage due to local invasion, rich vascularity, and the close relationship to great vessels. Many patients required coronary artery bypass grafting and invaded struc-tures reconstruction [6]. Cardiac transplantation has been suggested as a possible solution. Surgical risks particular to cardiac paragangliomas include fatal hemorrhage and hypertensive crisis related to intraoperative manipulation of the tumor. With reported recurrence rates of up to 25%, long-term imaging follow-up is recommended [3].

25.3   Current Technical Status and Applications of CT

CT is not first-line imaging modality generally but can often add significant information to the management of cardiac paraganglioma. These tumors are difficult to separate out from adjacent normal tissue. CT imaging is helpful to define the lesion anatomy and blood supply to aid surgical planning.

Multiphase ECG-gated CT imaging protocol is generally suggested for cardiac paraganglioma evaluation (including gated non-contrast, coronary CTA phase, and about 20-second delay phase). Multiphase scan can provide critical information about the extent and mobility of a cardiac mass and its effect on adjacent structures; coronary artery anatomy, patency, and relationship between coronary tree and the mass. ECG-gated cardiac CT examinations can be acquired using prospective or retrospective gating. Prospective gating has the advantage of significantly lower radiation doses, whereas retrospective gating offers the opportunity to reconstruct cine images evaluating valvular and cardiac function [7].

Tube current modulation and iterative reconstruction can be used to control the radiation dose. Dual-energy or perfusion techniques are selective, which extend the ability to include advanced tissue characterization and tumor blood supply [8]. Dual-energy CT (DECT) imaging can offer multiple postprocessing datasets with a single acquisition. The most commonly used DECT techniques for cardiac tumor include virtual non-contrast (VNC) imaging, iodine-enhanced image (iodine map), and automatic bone removal. Iodine concentration measurements with DECT data provide a reliable quantitative parameter to indicate lesion enhancement. VNC images may replace real non-contrast imaging to reduce radiation dose [9].

Advances in multi-detector CT hardware and sophisticated post-processing technique have made 3D reconstructions a useful adjunct for cardiac mass assessment. Maximum intensity projection (MIP) images are optimized for vascular anatomy evaluating and their relationship to the tumor. Volume rendering (VR) employs a more complex algorithm and allows for better visualization of soft tissues, bony structures, and vasculature in a single image. Cinematic rendering is a novel technique which is similar to VR but incorporates a more complex lighting model to create more photorealistic images to demarcate the margins and extent of tumor.

Three-dimensional printing using high-resolution CT data is useful for presurgical planning and the field is advancing rapidly. The additional value in a 3D model over a 3D reconstructed image has been largely attributed to easier visualization of the margins of the mass and a better appreciation of the relationship between the mass and the surrounding structures. It allows a surgeon to gain another level of insight by holding, turning, and manipulating a simulated model of the anatomy in question to help plan an operation before it begins [10]. For cardiac paraganglioma, its potential advantages are particularly obvious.

25.4 Key Points

- Primary cardiac paraganglioma is extremely rare but with classic characteristics. The diagnosis can be made on the basis of clinical information, biochemical lab tests, and nuclear medicine imaging.
- Contrast-enhanced CT is an essential complementary imaging technology to evaluate the lesion's range, blood supply, and anatomic relation to adjacent structures, which provide useful information to operation planning.
- Three-dimensional printing base on CT is an emerging technology which may offer additional value for cardiac paraganglioma operation.

References

1. Grebenc ML, Rosado de Christenson ML, Burke AP, Green CE, Galvin JR. Primary cardiac and pericardial neoplasms: radiologic-pathologic correlation. Radiographics. 2000;20(4):1073–103;. quiz 110-1, 112. https://doi.org/10.1148/radiographics.20.4.g00jl081073.
2. Araoz PA, Mulvagh SL, Tazelaar HD, Julsrud PR, Breen JF. CT and MR imaging of benign primary cardiac neoplasms with echocardiographic correlation. Radiographics. 2000;20(5):1303–19. https://doi.org/10.1148/radiographics.20.5.g00se121303.

3. El-Ashry AA, Cerfolio RJ, Singh SP, McGiffin D. Cardiac paraganglioma. J Card Surg. 2015;30(2):135–9. https://doi.org/10.1111/jocs.12479.

4. Almenieir N, Karls S, Derbekyan V, Lisbona R. Nuclear imaging of a cardiac paraganglioma. J Nucl Med Technol. 2017;45(3):247–8. https://doi.org/10.2967/jnmt.116.182212.

5. Manabe O, Oyama-Manabe N, Alisa K, Hirata K, Itoh K, Terae S, et al. Multimodality evaluation of cardiac paraganglioma. Clin Nucl Med. 2012;37(6):599–601. https://doi.org/10.1097/RLU.0b013e3182485204.

6. Khan MF, Datta S, Chisti MM, Movahed MR. Cardiac paraganglioma: clinical presentation, diagnostic approach and factors affecting short and long-term outcomes. Int J Cardiol. 2013;166(2):315–20. https://doi.org/10.1016/j.ijcard.2012.04.158.

7. Glockner JF. Magnetic resonance imaging and computed tomography of cardiac masses and pseudo-masses in the atrioventricular groove. Can Assoc Radiol J. 2018;69(1):78–91. https://doi.org/10.1016/j.carj.2017.12.004.

8. Young PM, Foley TA, Araoz PA, Williamson EE. Computed tomography imaging of cardiac masses. Radiol Clin N Am. 2019;57(1):75–84. https://doi.org/10.1016/j.rcl.2018.08.002.

9. Odisio EG, Truong MT, Duran C, de Groot PM, Godoy MC. Role of dual-energy computed tomography in thoracic oncology. Radiol Clin N Am. 2018;56(4):535–48. https://doi.org/10.1016/j.rcl.2018.03.011.

10. Liddy S, McQuade C, Walsh KP, Loo B, Buckley O. The assessment of cardiac masses by cardiac CT and CMR including pre-op 3D reconstruction and planning. Curr Cardiol Rep. 2019;21(9):103. https://doi.org/10.1007/s11886-019-1196-7.

Hypertrophic Cardiomyopathy

26

Yan Yi, Lu Lin, and Yining Wang

Abstract

Hypertrophic cardiomyopathy (HCM) is a relatively common disease that exhibits heterogeneous phenotypes with an autosomal dominant Mendelian pattern of inheritance. It is characterized by diverse phenotypic expressions and variable natural progression. Accurate diagnosis is of great importance for the perioperative management of these patients. Traditionally, the echocardiographic assessment and cardiac magnetic resonance imaging were both the methods of choice for evaluating HCM, which includes assessing the extent and location of left ventricular hypertrophy, left ventricular outflow tract gradients, systolic and diastolic function, anatomic as well as functional abnormalities of the mitral valve and papillary muscles. Recently, the rapid development of cardiac CT imaging technique provides more possibilities for its value in the differential diagnosis and condition evaluation of HCM patients. In this chapter, based on a case of apical HCM, we will discuss the cardiac CT imaging manifestations of HCM, and further possibly promising role of new cardiac CT technology in HCM.

Y. Yi · L. Lin · Y. Wang (✉)
Department of Radiology, Peking Union Medical College Hospital, Chinese Academy of Medical Sciences and Peking Union Medical College, Beijing, China
e-mail: wangyining@pumch.cn

26.1 Case of HCM

26.1.1 History

A 61-year-old male patient felt progressive exertional chest tightness which relieved by rest for the past 11 years. He had a recent dizziness in 10 days and appointed to cardiac CT for suspected coronary artery disease (CAD).

Physical Examination
- Blood pressure: 142/74 mm Hg; Breathing rate: 18/min; heart rate: 81 bpm without arrhythmia.
- 3/6 grade systolic murmurs are audible in the apical region

Electrocardiograph
Standard 12-lead electrocardiograph (ECG) revealed ST-T segment changes on leads V2–V6 and T wave inversion.

Laboratory
Serum myocardial enzyme spectrum showed negative results.

26.1.2 Imaging Examination

CT Images
A coronary CT angiography (CTA) combined with adenosine triphosphate (ATP)-stress myo-

© Springer Nature Singapore Pte Ltd. 2020
Z.-y. Jin et al. (eds.), *Cardiac CT*, https://doi.org/10.1007/978-981-15-5305-9_26

cardial CT perfusion was requested to investigate the coronary artery status and myocardial blood flow (Figs. 26.1, 26.2, and 26.3).

Conventional Coronary Angiography
See Fig. 26.4

26.1.3 Imaging Findings and Diagnosis

The coronary CTA images results showed there were mixed plaques in the proximal-middle segments of LAD and noncalcified plaques in the

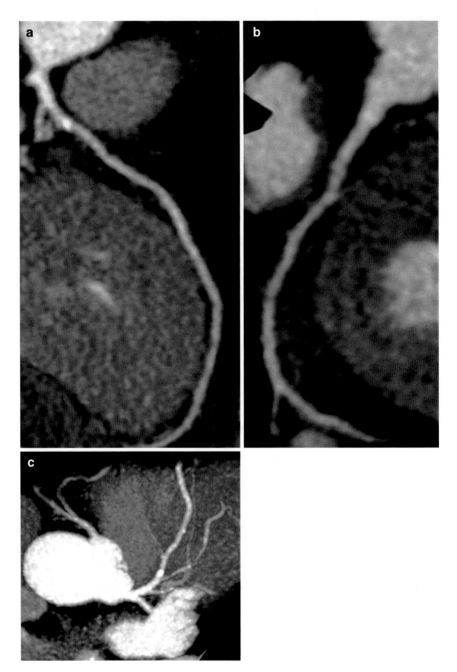

Fig. 26.1 Curved multi-planar (CPR) reconstructed images (**a**, left anterior descending [LAD] branch; **b**, left circumflex artery [LCx]) and thin maximum intensity pro-jection (MIP) image (**c**) of the coronary CTA. No signifi-cant stenosis has been shown in the three coronary arteries

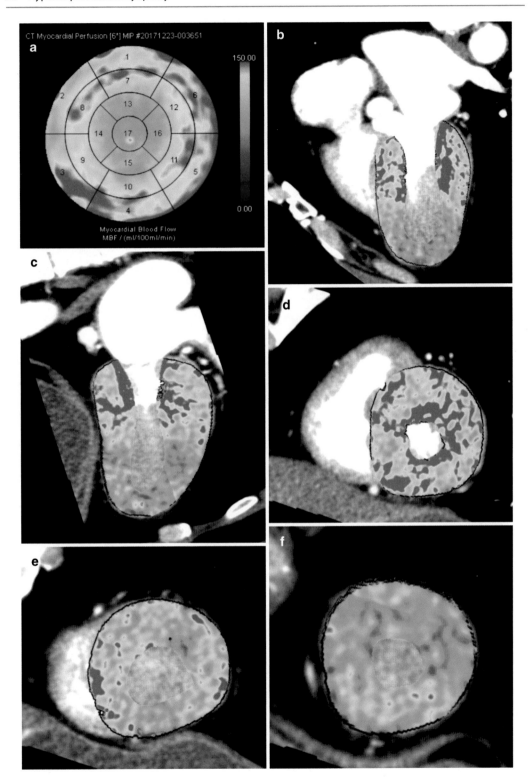

Fig. 26.2 CT perfusion myocardial blood flow (MBF) pseudo-color images: Bull-eye polar-map (**a**), four-chamber view (**b**), long-axis two-chamber view (**c**) and short-axis two-chamber views (**d-f**) of left ventricle showed an extensive MBF reduction in the periapical myocardium compared to the basal segments

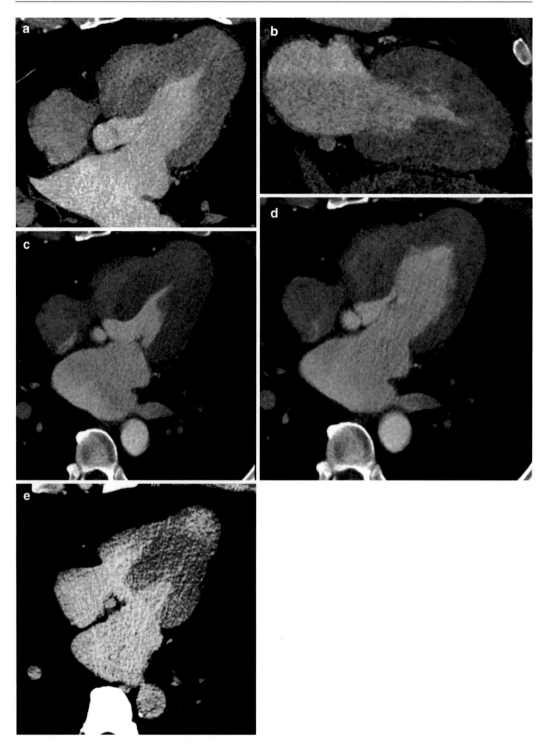

Fig. 26.3 Cardiac CT imaging of myocardium: four-chamber view (**a**) and long-axis two-chamber view (**b**) of left ventricular. Delayed scan imaging of long-axis views in the systolic phase (**c**, MPR image; **e**, dual-energy iodine maps) and diastolic phase (**d**) showed a thickened apical myocardium with partially patchy mid-wall delayed enhancement

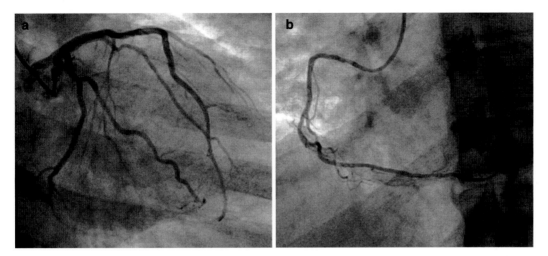

Fig. 26.4 Percutaneous transluminal coronary intervention (PCI) results. Invasive coronary angiography image for LAD (**a**), LCX (**a**) and right coronary artery (RCA) (**b**), confirmed no significant stenosis in the coronary arteries

proximal-middle segments of LCX, resulting in both mild lumen stenosis. No significant stenosis has been found in all the coronary arteries. All the myocardial perfusion of left ventricular (LV) images, including bull-eye polar-maps, four-chamber views, two-long chamber views, and two-short chamber views, showed the extensive reduction of myocardial blood flow in apical portion compared to the basal area, which do not correspond to the coronary blood supply region of lesion vessels. The four-chamber views and two-long chamber views of both systolic and diastolic LV delayed CT scan results show a thickened apical myocardium. Partially in the delayed phase of dual-energy iodine maps, the apparent enhancement of the apical portion suggested local fibrosis. The invasive coronary angiography images confirmed only several mild stenosis on the LAD and RCA.

26.1.4 Management

- Conventional medical therapy for Secondary Prevention of CAD
- Out-patient follow-up observations for HCM

26.2 Discussion

HCM is one of the most common monogenic cardiovascular disorders, affecting 1 of every 500 adults. It is characterized by diverse phenotypic expressions, including focal basal septum HCM, diffuse septum HCM, concentric and diffuse HCM, burned-out phase HCM, mid-ventricular HCM, apical HCM, focal mid-septum HCM, free-wall HCM, and crypts in genotype-positive and phenotype-negative HCM.

The asymmetric septal form is the most common morphologic variant of HCM and accounts for up to 60–70% of cases [1]. It is typically presented with the disproportionate enlargement of the ventricular septum, with the anteroseptal myocardium most commonly involved. The diagnostic criteria consist of basal septal thickness ≥15 mm; the ratio of septal thickness to thickness of inferior wall at mid-ventricular level >1.5.

The symmetrical or concentric HCM ranked the second most common phenotype and is characterized by diffuse left ventricular wall thickening with an associated decrease in left ventricular cavity size [1, 2]. Diagnosis should be made in the absence of a secondary cause like hypertension, aortic stenosis, or the patient being an endurance athlete.

Apical HCM accounts for approximately 2–15% of all the HCM cases [1, 3]. It is typically presented with giant negative T waves on the electrocardiogram and a spade-like configuration of the LV cavity, which resulted from the apical portion hypertrophy of the LV. Diagnosis of the apical HCM depends on LV thickening (predominantly confined to the apex measuring 15 mm or more) and the ratio of apical LV wall thicknesses to basal LV wall thicknesses (1.3–1.5) [1].

Clinically, patients with apical HCM may present with exertional angina or dyspnea and may have electrocardiographic findings similar to those with CAD or in acute coronary syndromes [1, 4]. Differential diagnosis is important.

26.3 Current Technical Status and Applications of CT

Although cardiac MR imaging has advantages for accurate diagnosis, Cardiac Computed Tomographic (CT) scan technology has showed a complementary role for these patients [3, 5–7]. Cardiac CT is able to identify the hypertrophy of the myocardium and as well as the asymmetry of the ventricular hypertrophy [7, 8]. When a 4D cardiac CT imaging was performed, the left ventricular outflow tract obstruction (LVOTO) and the mitral valve and papillary muscles situation can be clearly showed with a dynamic imaging as MR [9]. The geometric predictors of LVOTO measured by cardiac CT in HCM patients have been demonstrated as independent predictors, including Spiral pattern of LV hypertrophy, the length of the anterior mitral leaflet (AML), and the distance between lateral papillary muscle (PM) base and left ventricular (LV) apex [10]. Furthermore, the CT angiography planning improves the localization of infarct and procedural success at the first attempt in Alcohol septal ablation (ASA) when compared

to traditional methods. Follow-up to 6 months suggests a symptomatic, functional, and hemodynamic improvement [11]. Besides, the cardiac CT is possibly contributing for revealing the enlarged mitral valve and systolic anterior motion (SAM) of the mitral valve or mitral valve regurgitation [8].

Some of these HCM patients were admitted for PCI because of suspected CAD. A coronary CTA is always clinically referred for before the invasive angiography. Recently, with the rapid development of CT technology, the perfusion imaging approach has become more and more prevalent in the clinical application. Coronary CTA combined with ATP-stress myocardial CT perfusion can be organized as pre-opreative examination to investigate the coronary artery stenosis and myocardial blood flow. Mild lumen stenosis and unmatched local extensive reduction of myocardial blood flow combined with myocardium thickness on Cardiac CT can highly suggest the diagnosis of HCM [1, 3, 4]. Apart from apical hypertrophy, other atypical forms of HCM including concentric hypertrophy or sometimes mid-ventricular hypertrophy can also be demonstrated by CT imaging [8].

In addition, dual-energy cardiac CT imaging can be utilized for a delayed scan of the HCM patients. The delayed enhancement mostly focal but can be diffuse, which is particularly obvious in the iodine maps, suggesting fibrosis of the myocardium. It can be related to life-threatening arrhythmia and cardiac death [4, 8].

Lately, the fractional flow reserve derived from CT (FFRCT) has shown its potential value for HCM patients. It offers a noninvasive method for evaluating the coronary artery volume to myocardial mass ratio (V/M), which demonstrated significantly greater coronary volume yet decreased V/M for HCM patients [12].

Appropriate cardiac CT examination contributes a lot for correct differential diagnosis thinking and prompt treatment choice, as well as accurate prognosis assessment.

26.4 Key Points

- HCM may present with exertional angina or dyspnea, or have electrocardiographic findings similar to those with CAD or in acute coronary syndromes.
- Appropriate cardiac CT examination with developing imaging technologies may contribute to correct differential diagnosis of HCM from CAD and myocardial viability and fibrosis evaluation.

References

1. Baxi AJ, Restrepo CS, Vargas D, et al. Hypertrophic cardiomyopathy from A to Z: genetics, pathophysiology, imaging, and management. Radiographics. 2016;36(2):335–54.
2. Hansen MW, Merchant N. MRI of hypertrophic cardiomyopathy: part I, MRI appearances. AJR Am J Roentgenol. 2007;189(6):1335–43.
3. Maron BJ, Maron MS. Hypertrophic cardiomyopathy. Lancet. 2013;381(9862):242–55.
4. Ho CY, Lopez B, Coelho-Filho OR, et al. Myocardial fibrosis as an early manifestation of hypertrophic cardiomyopathy. N Engl J Med. 2010;363(6):552–63.
5. Brouwer WP, Baars EN, Germans T, et al. In-vivo T1 cardiovascular magnetic resonance study of diffuse myocardial fibrosis in hypertrophic cardiomyopathy. J Cardiovasc Magn Reson. 2014;16:28.
6. Maron MS. Clinical utility of cardiovascular magnetic resonance in hypertrophic cardiomyopathy. J Cardiovasc Magn Reson. 2012;14:13.
7. Rickers C, Wilke NM, Jerosch-Herold M, et al. Utility of cardiac magnetic resonance imaging in the diagnosis of hypertrophic cardiomyopathy. Circulation. 2005;112(6):855–61.
8. Khalil H, Alzahrani T. Cardiomyopathy imaging. Treasure Island, FL: StatPearls; 2019.
9. Rajiah P, Fulton NL, Bolen M. Magnetic resonance imaging of the papillary muscles of the left ventricle: normal anatomy, variants, and abnormalities. Insights. Imaging. 2019;10(1):83.
10. Song Y, Yang DH, Harrtaigh BO, et al. Geometric predictors of left ventricular outflow tract obstruction in patients with hypertrophic cardiomyopathy: a 3D computed tomography analysis. Eur Heart J Cardiovasc Imaging. 2018;19(10):1149–56.
11. Cooper RM, Binukrishnan SR, Shahzad A, et al. Computed tomography angiography planning identifies the target vessel for optimum infarct location and improves clinical outcome in alcohol septal ablation for hypertrophic obstructive cardiomyopathy. EuroIntervention. 2017;12(18):e2194–203.
12. Sellers SL, Fonte TA, Grover R, et al. Hypertrophic Cardiomyopathy (HCM): New insights into Coronary artery remodelling and ischemia from FFRCT. J Cardiovasc Comput Tomogr. 2018;12(6):467–71.

Dilated Cardiomyopathy

27

Fan Yang, Zhang Zhang, and Dong Li

Abstract

Dilated cardiomyopathy (DCM) is character-ized by left ventricle (LV) or biventricular dilatation and systolic dysfunction without overloading conditions and predominantly affects younger adults. Though the etiology is various, Computed Tomographic (CT) could evaluate the degree of LV dilatation and con-tractile impairment which is the major deter-minant of prognosis. Although cardiac magnetic resonance (MR) imaging has an advantage in diagnosis DCM, cardiac CT can detect abnormal chambers, myocardium, and cardiac function and assist to except coronary artery disease and valvular abnormality within a short scanning time. Additionally, the advanced CT imaging technique could offer more information about DCM patients. In this chapter, based on the case of typical DCM, we will discuss the basic and new CT perfor-mance of DCM.

27.1 Case of DCM

27.1.1 History

- A 32-year-old male patient felt progressive exertional chest tightness and dyspnea which relieved by rest for the past 3 months.
- His symptom exacerbated with a recent hemoptysis in 2 days.

Physical Examination
- Blood pressure: 119/93 mm Hg; Breathing rate: 22/min
- Heart rate: 97 bpm without arrhythmia and murmurs

Electrocardiograph
- Non-sustained ventricular tachycardia within 24 h.

Laboratory
- Serum myocardial enzyme spectrum showed negative results.
- NTpro-BNP result revealed up to 2455 pg/ml.

27.1.2 Imaging Examination

CT Images
A coronary CT angiography (CTA) was acquired to investigate the coronary artery (Figs. 27.1, 27.2, 27.3, and 27.4).

F. Yang · Z. Zhang · D. Li (✉)
Radiology Department, Tianjin Medical University General Hospital, Tianjin, China

© Springer Nature Singapore Pte Ltd. 2020
Z.-y. Jin et al. (eds.), *Cardiac CT*, https://doi.org/10.1007/978-981-15-5305-9_27

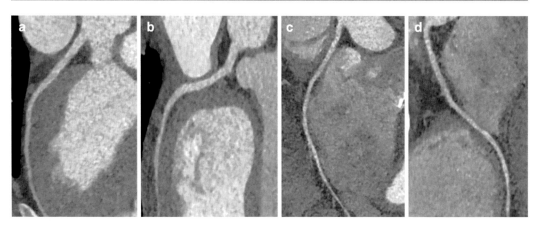

Fig. 27.1 Curved multi-planar (CPR) reconstructed images of (**a**) left anterior descending (LAD), (**b**) left circumflex artery (LCX), (**c**) right coronary artery (RCA) and (**d**) posterior descending artery (PDA) from the coronary CTA. No significant stenosis and plaque have been shown in the coronary arteries

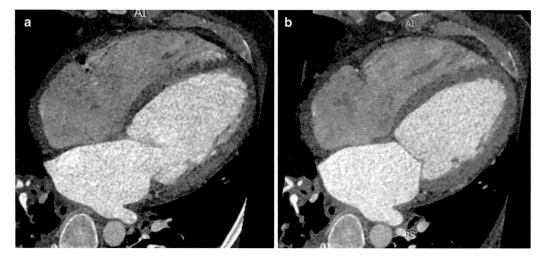

Fig. 27.2 Cardiac CT imaging of myocardium on four-chamber view in diastolic phase (**a**) and systolic phase (**b**) also showed dilated spherical-like left ventricle and decreased systolic function. Left atrium and right ventricle were also slightly dilated

27.1.3 Imaging Findings and Diagnosis

The coronary CTA images results showed there were no plaques and lumen stenosis in the coronary arteries. Cardiac reconstructions, including four-chamber views, two-chamber views, three-chamber views, and short-axial views, showed extensive dilatation and declined systolic wall thickening associated with low systolic function of the left ventricle. Furthermore, the left atrium and right ventricle were slightly dilated. Additionally, the two-chamber views, three-chamber views, and four-chamber views results showed no thickened or regurgitation on the mitral valve and aortic valve. Pericardial effusion is detected.

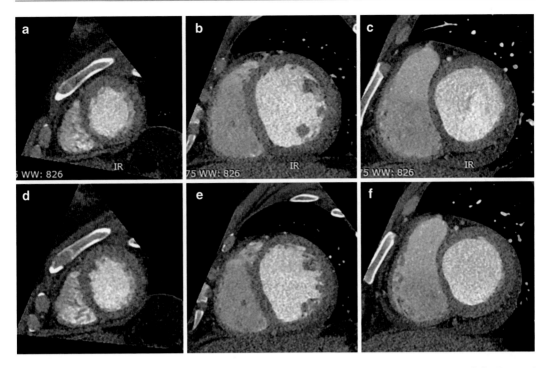

Fig. 27.3 Cardiac CT short-axial multi-planer reconstructed images of diastolic (**a–c**) and systolic (**d–f**) phases of ventricles showed dilated left ventricle and decreased systolic wall thickening as well as pericardial effusion

27.1.4 Management

- Diuretic and cardiotonic therapy for improving cardiac function.
- Out-patient follow-up observations for DCM and heart failure.

27.2   Discussion

DCM is currently defined by the performance of LV or biventricular dilatation and systolic dysfunction without coronary artery disease or abnormal loading conditions (hypertension, valvular heart disease, and so on.) sufficient to cause global systolic impairment. DCM predominantly affects younger adults. The etiology can be genetic or nongenetic including toxins, infectious, endocrine, inflammatory, neuromuscular disease, and others [1, 2]. The differential diagnosis of the causes is important and may be helpful for inter-

vention, because DCM is the most frequent indication for cardiac transplantation. The assessment of the degree of LV dilatation, systolic dysfunction, and myocardial fibrosis in DCM is the dominating determinant of adverse outcomes.

The diagnostic criteria of DCM consist of reduced ejection fraction (EF < 45%) and LV dilatation. LV dilatation is defined as LV end-diastolic volumes (EDV) or diameters >2SD from normal according to normograms [1]. However, a number of patients developed presymptomatic DCM who have subtle or minimal myocardial injury, dysfunction, or remodeling. Early intervention can slow down adverse remodeling, prevent heart failure, and increase life expectancy.

Clinically, patients with DCM may present with exertional angina or dyspnea and may similar to those with other diseases presented as heart failure. We also should be wary of youth patients who present atypical symptoms.

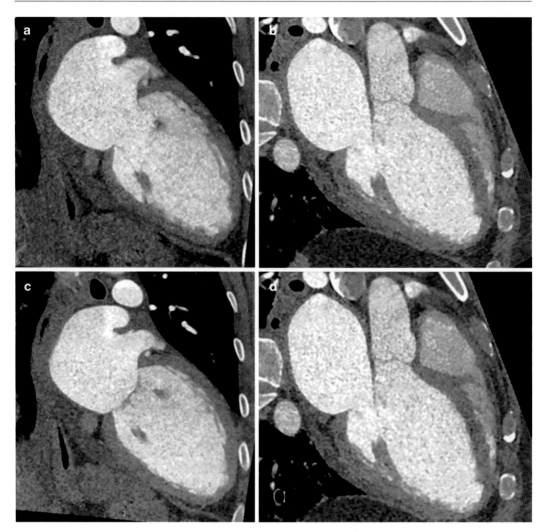

Fig. 27.4 Cardiac CT imaging of myocardium on long axial views of left ventricular (**a**, **c**) and three-chamber views (**b**, **d**) in diastolic (**a**, **b**) and systolic phases (**c**, **d**) detected dilated left ventricle without abnormalities in mitral valve and aortic valve. Left atrium was slightly dilated

27.3   Current Technical Status and Applications of CT

Although cardiac MR imaging has obvious privilege for accurate diagnosis DCM, Cardiac Computed Tomographic (CT) can assist to except coronary artery disease and valvular abnormality. Furthermore, Cardiac CT is able to identify the dilated ventricle and the associated remodeling of the whole heart. Actually, cardiac CT offers several advantages over MR, including obtaining the whole myocardium in a short scanning time, and widespread availability, even substituted for cardiac MR in case of MR contraindications.

After contrast injection, excellent delineation of the blood–myocardium interface enables to assess the volume and diameter of chambers. Left atrial (LA) dilatation is frequently detected in DCM as a consequence of LV diastolic impairment and enlargement; LA volume is valuable for predicting adverse outcomes in DCM [3]. Pulmonary hypertension and secondary adverse right ventricular (RV) remodeling is also common in DCM patients. These indices provide independent prognostic information in DCM. Besides, CT may be contributing for performing the associated enlarged mitral valve.

In recent years, dual-energy CT imaging technology has become more and more prevalent in the clinical application as well as in myocardial tissue characteristics. Dual-energy cardiac CT can be utilized for investigating the delayed contrast enhancement and extracellular volume (ECV) fraction. CT ECV map depicted ECV on a color-coded map and correlated well with late gadolinium enhancement (LGE) of CMR, which is typically in the mid myocardium of interventricular septum, suggesting fibrosis of the myocardium [4, 5]. Additionally, myocardial perfusion CT is able to evaluate intramyocardial microcirculation in DCM.

Advanced cardiac CT examination could provide multiple aspects of DCM patients and as well as accurate prognosis assessment.

27.4 Key Points

- DCM patients may present with atypical symptoms and electrocardiographic findings and hospitalize for heart failure at initial consultation.
- Cardiac CT examination may contribute to correct differential diagnosis of DCM from CAD and valvular heart disease.

References

1. Pinto YM, Elliott PM, Arbustini E, et al. Proposal for a revised definition of dilated cardiomyopathy, hypokinetic non-dilated cardiomyopathy, and its implications for clinical practice: A position statement of the ESC working group on myocardial and pericardial diseases. Eur Heart J. 2016;37(23):1850–8.
2. Japp AG, Gulati A, Cook SA, et al. The diagnosis and evaluation of dilated cardiomyopathy. J Am Coll Cardiol. 2016;67(25):2996–3010.
3. Gulati A, Ismail TF, Jabbour A, et al. Clinical utility and prognostic value of left atrial volume assessment by cardiovascular magnetic resonance in non-ischaemic dilated cardiomyopathy. Eur J Heart Fail. 2013;15(6):660–70.
4. Cerny V, Kuchynka P, Marek J, et al. Utility of cardiac CT for evaluating delayed contrast enhancement in dilated cardiomyopathy. Herz. 2017;42(8):776–80.
5. Hong YJ, Kim TK, Hong D, et al. Myocardial characterization using dual-energy CT in doxorubicin-induced DCM: comparison with CMR T1-mapping and histology in a rabbit model. JACC Cardiovasc Imaging. 2016;9(7):836–45.

Restrictive Cardiomyopathy

28

Xiao Li and Yining Wang

Abstract

Restrictive cardiomyopathy (RCM) is a relatively rare myocardial disorder characterized as increased myocardial stiffness that leads to diastolic dysfunction. Biventricular chamber size and systolic function are usually normal or near-normal until later stages of the disease. Patients may have signs or symptoms of left or/and right heart failure. RCM is a heterogeneous group that is broadly classified as infiltrative, storage disease, noninfiltrative, and endomyocardial. Accurate diagnosis is of great importance. Echocardiography can be the first imaging modality to evaluate ventricular dysfunction. Cardiac MRI is the optimal imaging modality, providing one-stop, multiparameter evaluation of cardiac chamber size, diastolic dysfunction, the presence of myocardial fibrosis, and differentiation from other causes of cardiomyopathy. CT plays a complementary role to differential diagnosis thinking and treatment choice, as well as prognosis assessment. In this chapter, based

on a case of Löffler endocarditis, we will discuss the cardiac CT imaging manifestations of RCM, and further possibly promising role of new cardiac CT technology in RCM.

28.1 Case of RCM

28.1.1 History

A 45-year-old man was hospitalized with recurrent cough and left chest pain for 6 months. The peripheral blood count revealed a marked hypereosinophilia (52.3%).

28.1.2 Imaging Examination

CT Images
See Figs. 28.1 and 28.2.

MRI Images
See Figs. 28.3 and 28.4.

28.1.3 Imaging Findings and Diagnosis

Contrast-enhanced CT showed the left ventricle was enlarged, and the apical wall of the left ventricle was thickened with a "peach-shaped" appearance. There was an irregular, mural, and

X. Li · Y. Wang (✉)
Department of Radiology, Peking Union Medical College Hospital, Chinese Academy of Medical Sciences and Peking Union Medical College, Beijing, China
e-mail: wangyining@pumch.cn

© Springer Nature Singapore Pte Ltd. 2020
Z.-y. Jin et al. (eds.), *Cardiac CT*, https://doi.org/10.1007/978-981-15-5305-9_28

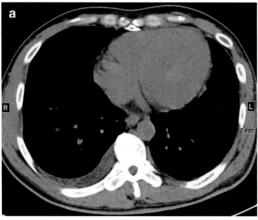
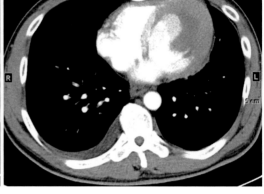

Fig. 28.1 Plain scan (**a**) and contrast-enhanced (**b**) CT showed the left ventricle was enlarged, and the apical wall of the left ventricle was thickened with a "peach-shaped" appearance. There was an irregular, mural, and slightly high density without enhancement in the left ventricle chamber

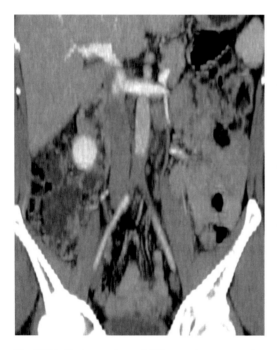

Fig. 28.2 Contrast-enhanced CT coronal reconstruction image showed a focal filling defect in the distal segment of the abdominal aorta and bilateral common iliac artery

slightly high density without enhancement in the left ventricle chamber. Coronal reconstruction image showed a focal filling defect in the distal segment of the abdominal aorta and bilateral common iliac artery. Cardiac magnetic resonance cine image showed the left atrium and left ventricle were enlarged, with restrictive

diastolic dysfunction and preserved ejection fraction (64.3%). The apical wall of the left ventricle was thickened with a "peach-shaped" appearance. Dynamic gadolinium-enhanced scan showed a predominantly subendocardial, focal transmural decrease of first-pass perfusion and late gadolinium enhancement of the septum and left ventricle. There was a mural, non-enhanced signal in the left ventricle chamber. Native T1 map, T2 map, and extracellular volume map revealed a mildly increased global value of 1373 ms, 42 ms, and 36%, respectively. A diagnosis of Löffler endocarditis with thrombosis was made.

28.1.4 Management

- The patient received a standard therapy of prednisone.
- Three months later as the level of eosinophils turned normal, the patient received aortic valve replacement, thrombectomy, and endocardectomy. During the surgery, the endocardium of the septum and the apical segment of the left ventricle were found to be diffusely thickened and fibrotic.
- Biopsy confirmed a coarse endocardium with organized thrombosis, as well as myocardium degeneration and fibrosis with chronic inflammatory infiltration.

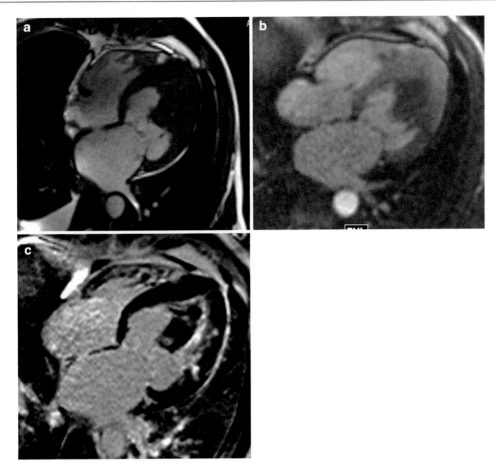

Fig. 28.3 Cardiac magnetic resonance cine image (**a**) showed the left atrium and left ventricle were enlarged, with restrictive diastolic dysfunction and preserved ejection fraction (64.3%). The apical wall of the left ventricle was thickened with a "peach-shaped" appearance. Dynamic gadolinium-enhanced scan showed a predominantly subendocardial, focal transmural decrease of first-pass perfusion (**b**) and late gadolinium enhancement of the septum and left ventricle (**c**). There was a mural, non-enhanced signal in the left ventricle chamber

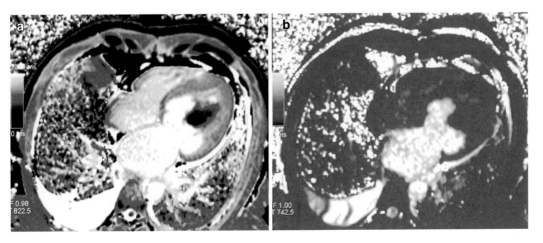

Fig. 28.4 Cardiac magnetic resonance Native T1 map (**a**), T2 map (**b**) and extracellular volume map (**c**) revealed a mildly increased global value of 1373 ms, 42 ms, and 36%, respectively

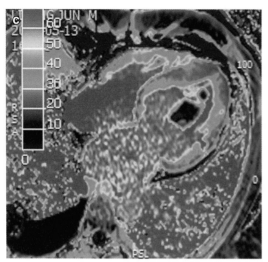

Fig. 28.4 (continued)

28.2 Discussion

RCM is a relatively rare myocardial disorder characterized as increased myocardial stiffness that leads to diastolic dysfunction. Biventricular chamber size and systolic function are usually normal or near-normal until later stages of the disease [1]. Patients may have signs or symptoms of left or/and right heart failure [2].

RCM is a heterogeneous group that varies according to pathogenesis, clinical presentation, diagnostic evaluation and criteria, treatment, and prognosis, which is broadly classified as infiltrative, storage disease, noninfiltrative, and endomyocardial [1].

Amyloidosis is an infiltrative disease of extracellular deposition of amyloid insoluble proteins in the heart and other tissues or/and organs. Characteristic imaging findings include thickening of the ventricular and atrial walls as well as the interatrial septum. Echocardiography depicts speckled appearance of the myocardium. MRI typically shows global, predominantly subendocardial late enhancement [3].

Hereditary hemochromatosis is classified as a storage disease caused by iron deposition in various organs and tissues. Cardiac involvement is uncommon. Characteristic imaging findings include decreased myocardial signal intensity in T1-, T2-, and T2*-weighted images, and decreased myocardial global value in T1, T2, and T2* maps [4, 5].

Hypereosinophilic syndrome is classified as extensive endomyocardial fibrosis of the subendocardial layer of the myocardium involving the apices and extending to the inflow tracts. Characteristic imaging findings include thickened, predominantly apical ventricular wall, and enlarged atrial chamber. Thrombus formation is common and may obliterate the entire ventricular apex. MRI depicts subendocardial delayed enhancement [6].

Idiopathic RCM is characterized as restrictive physiology in the absence of any identifiable cause. Patients may have certain genetic mutations and family history [1].

Treatment and prognosis of RCM vary depending on etiology. Medical management of heart failure, anticoagulation for patients at risk of thromboembolic events, and heart transplantation may be performed if necessary [2].

28.3 Current Technical Status and Applications of CT

Echocardiography can be the first imaging modality to evaluate ventricular dysfunction. At early presentation, radiographic findings may be normal, or impaired diastolic function is seen with atrial enlargement. Later stage demonstrates impaired systolic function or elevated pulmonary arterial pressure. Cardiac MRI is the optimal imaging modality, providing one-stop, multiparameter evaluation of cardiac chamber size, diastolic dysfunction, the presence of myocardial fibrosis, and differentiation from other causes of cardiomyopathy [4].

CT is nonspecific for restrictive cardiomyopathy but can play a complementary role. Cardiac CT is able to identify the primary and secondary morphological and histological changes, such as cardiac chamber enlargement, wall thinning and thickening, myocardial fat infiltration, and calcification [4, 5]. 4D cardiac CT enables functional evaluation as dynamic MRI. Dual-energy cardiac CT imaging can be utilized for a delayed scan, and depict delayed enhancement in the iodine maps, suggesting myocardial fibrosis.

CT examination contributes to differential diagnosis thinking and treatment choice, as well as prognosis assessment. CT helps in delineating mediastinal and hilar adenopathy with calcifications in sarcoidosis, thrombosis in hypereosinophilic syndrome as well as associated lung findings, and pericardial thickening, calcification, and cardiac morphological changes in constrictive pericarditis [4, 5]. A coronary CT angiography is always clinically referred to exclude coronary arterial disease and myocardial infarction.

28.4 Key Points

- RCM is a relatively rare myocardial disorder characterized as increased myocardial stiffness that leads to diastolic dysfunction.
- RCM is a heterogeneous group that broadly classified as infiltrative, storage disease, noninfiltrative, and endomyocardial.

- Echocardiography and MRI are first-line imaging modality.
- CT plays a complementary role to differential diagnosis thinking and treatment choice, as well as prognosis assessment.

References

1. Muchtar E, Blauwet LA, Gertz MA. Restrictive cardiomyopathy genetics, pathogenesis, clinical manifestations, diagnosis, and therapy. Circ Res. 2017;121:819–37.
2. McLaughlin DP, Stouffer GA. Cardiovascular hemodynamics for the clinician. Second ed. New York: Wiley; 2017. p. 212–7.
3. Fontana M, Pica S, Reant P, Abdel-Gadir A, et al. Prognostic value of late gadolinium enhancement cardiovascular magnetic resonance in cardiac amyloidosis. Circulation. 2015;132(16):1570–9.
4. Kim YJ, Choi BW. Practical textbook of cardiac CT and MRI. Berlin, Heidelberg: Springer; 2015. p. 199–206.
5. McCourt J, Richardson RR. Atlas of acquired cardiovascular disease imaging in children. Cham, Switzerland: Springer; 2017. p. 147–50.
6. Katre RS, Sunnapwar A, Restrepo CS, et al. Cardiopulmonary and gastrointestinal manifestations of eosinophil-associated diseases and idiopathic hypereosinophilic syndromes: multimodality imaging approach. RadioGraphics. 2016;36:433–51.

Arrhythmogenic Right Ventricular Cardiomyopathy

29

Jian Wang, Yining Wang, and Zheng-yu Jin

Abstract

Arrhythmogenic right ventricular cardiomy-opathy (ARVC) is a kind of inherited cardio-myopathy that predominantly affects the right ventricle. Although early detection and treat-ment is of vital importance, the diagnosis of ARVC right now remains challenging. Current task force criteria specify a series of diagnos-tic major and minor criteria in six categories. Among all right ventricle imaging methods, echocardiography (echo) and cardiac mag-netic resonance (CMR) are of vital importance for ARVC diagnosis. In this chapter, based on a case of ARVE, we will discuss the multimo-dality of imaging method in diagnosis of ARVC.

29.1 Case of ARVC

29.1.1 History

A 36-year-old female had shortness of breath and chest pain, with edema of lower limbs for more than 11 months.

J. Wang · Y. Wang · Z.-y. Jin (✉)
Department of Radiology, Peking Union Medical College Hospital, Chinese Academy of Medical Sciences and Peking Union Medical College, Beijing, China
e-mail: jinzy@pumch.cn

Physical Examination
- Blood pressure: 106/66 mm Hg; Breathing rate: 16/min
- Heart rate: 80 bpm without arrhythmia; aus-cultation with no murmur

Electrocardiograph

Standard 12-lead electrocardiograph (ECG) revealed sinus rhythm, low limb conduction voltage, incomplete right bundle branch block. V1–V3 leads have Epsilon waves, with T wave inversion.

Holter
- Sinus rhythm
- Frequent atrial premature, partial paired, short atrial tachycardia (410 times/24 h)
- Sporadic polygenic ventricular premature beats, partial pairings, and diploidy (1218 beats/24 h)
- Incomplete right bundle branch block

Laboratory
- NT-proBNP 738 pg/mL.
- Other serum myocardial enzyme spectrum showed negative results.

Family History

The patient's father passed away due to cardiac disease at the age of 41.

Z.-y. Jin et al. (eds.), *Cardiac CT*, https://doi.org/10.1007/978-981-15-5305-9_29

29.1.2 Imaging Examination

CT Images
A coronary CT angiography (CTA) was requested to investigate the coronary artery and the cardiac morphology (Fig. 29.1).

Echocardiography
Right heart enlargement with tricuspid valve severely incompletely closed. Systolic function of the right ventricle (RV) decreased. No pericardial fluid.

Cardiac Magnetic Resonance (CMR)
A CMR was requested to evaluate the cardiac morphology (Fig 29.2).

29.1.3 Imaging Findings and Diagnosis

The coronary CTA images showed no significant stenosis among the LCX, LAD, and RCA. RA and RV were enlarged, with a small amount of pericardial effusion.

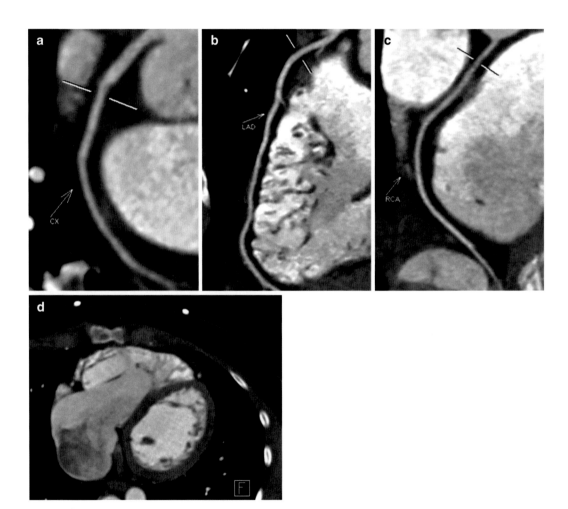

Fig. 29.1 (a–c) Curved multi-planar (CPR) of reconstructed images, (a, left circumflex artery, LCX, b, left anterior descending artery, LAD, c, right coronary artery) (d) axial view of the right atrium (RA), left ventricle (LV), right ventricle (RV). No significant stenosis has been shown in the three coronary arteries, and right atrium and right ventricle enlargement

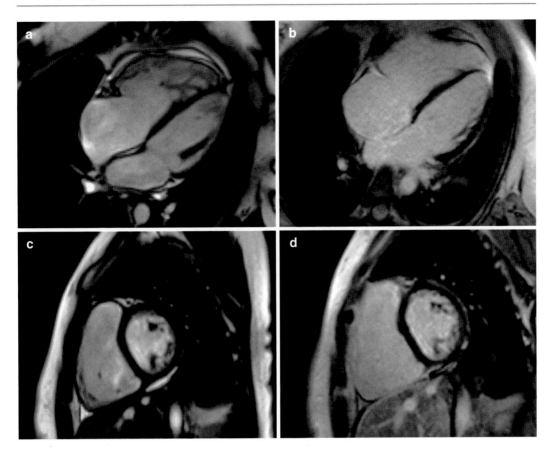

Fig. 29.2 (a) Four-chamber view of cine sequence at the end of diastolic, (b) four-chamber view of delayed enhancement, (c) basal of short axis of sequence at the end of diastolic, (d) basal of short axis of delayed enhancement

Echocardiography showed right heart enlargement with severe tricuspid valve regurgitation. Systolic function of RV decreased. No pericardial fluid.

The CMR showed RA and RV enlargement with tricuspid regurgitation, widening of the right ventricle outflow tract and increased RV trabecular porosity, with segmental decreased RV free wall contraction. RVEF = 41.9%. Left ventricle (LV) systolic motion decrease: LVEF = 46.3%. Small amount of pericardial effusion could be found. Fat-like signal can be observed in the interatrial septum. Suspicious gadolinium delayed enhancement emerged in the mid-wall of the ventricular septum.

According to the 2010 task force criteria, the diagnostic criteria are set as two major criteria or

one major with two minor criteria or four minor criteria. The patient meets three major criteria (① ECG abnormal depolarization; ② ECG abnormal repolarization; ③ diffuse or local dysfunction and structural changes), and 1 minor criteria (family history of cardiac disease). The patient can be diagnosed as ARVC.

29.1.4 Management

- Strictly control the amount of input and output, monitor ECG, be aware of fatal arrhythmia and sudden death.
- Regularly reexamination of echo, adjust drug dose, and run gene test if necessary.

29.2 Discussion

Arrhythmogenic right ventricular cardiomyopathy (ARVC) is an inherited cardiomyopathy that predominantly affects the right ventricle. The genetic basis of disease primarily involves in the cardiac desmosomes. The prevalence of ARVC is estimated between 1:5000 and 1:2000. It is one of the major causes of ventricular arrhythmia, congestive heart failure, and sudden death in young people and athletes [1].

The main characteristic histopathological feature of ARVC is replacing the normal right ventricular myocardial tissue with fibro-fatty tissue. This process proceeds from epicardium to endocardium, and finally results in wall thinning and aneurysmal dilatation. The typical "triangle of dysplasia" of ARVC includes ① inflow tract, ② outflow tract, and ③ apex of the right ventricle.

There is no single image finding which can direct pathognomonic diagnose for ARVC. Currently, the 2010 task force criteria are used in clinic, which classified as major criteria and minor criteria, and totally have six categories [2]. Different diagnostic modalities' findings must be combined and establish as "define," "borderline," or "possible" as diagnosis of ARVC.

Echocardiography (echo) is currently the first-line imaging modality to diagnose ARVC. The 2010 task force criteria also include CMR, which can provide a more accurate and reproducible measurement of each chamber dimension volumes and function [3]. As the anatomy complexity and load dependency in ARVC, discrepancy between echo and CMR have been observed; only 50% of patients fulfilled CMR criteria also satisfying the echo criteria [4].

Multidetector CT (MDCT) can be used to evaluate fatty tissue in right ventricular, as well as left ventricular, but compared to CMR the potential limitation of MDCT is the absence of function evaluation and the radiation dose, especially when assessing cardiac motion over the whole cardiac cycle. However, CT is feasible and useful in patients with ICD implants and has contraindications to CMR.

29.3 Current Technical Status and Applications of CT

Although cardiac MR imaging has advantages for accurate diagnosis, Cardiac CT scan technology has shown a complementary role for these patients. ECG-gated MDCT has lower temporal resolution and higher spatial resolution to MR imaging. Although in the 2010 task force criteria, the presence of RV myocardial fat is not the requirement for diagnose, but the fatty replacement of RV myocardium with free wall thinning could be considered as a characteristic finding of ARVC [5], especially in young patients, because the presence of fatty tissue in the right ventricle or interventricular septum or both areas are very helpful for diagnosing ARVC, as physiologic myocardial fat is more abundant with aged people. Unenhanced CT images enable to detect myocardial fat, while enhanced CT images permit to evaluate of the enlargement of the RV outflow tract and RV body, located fatty tissue, and thinning wall as well as bulging of the RV free wall [6].

In addition, overreliance detailed on CT finding of structural abnormality and myocardial fatty tissue may lead to a false-positive diagnosis. RV dilatation is observed in many kinds of cardiac diseases, such as some valvular heart diseases, congenital heart diseases, chronic pulmonary diseases, and dilated cardiomyopathy.

29.4 Key Points

- ARVC is an inherited disease, manifested as a gradual enlargement of the right ventricle, thinning of the RV free wall, and gradual cardiac tissue replacement with fatty tissue, which can cause fatal arrhythmia.
- Echo and CMR are essential imaging modalities for the diagnosis of ARVC.
- Cardiac CT is a good supplement examination, which can identify cardiac morphology and fat tissue in high temporal resolution.

References

1. Bhonsale A, Groeneweg JA, James CA, Dooijes D, Tichnell C, Jongbloed JD, et al. Impact of genotype on clinical course in arrhythmogenic right ventricular dysplasia/cardiomyopathy-associated mutation carriers. Eur Heart J. 2015;36(14):847.

2. Peters MN, Katz MJ, MEJP A. Diagnosis of arrhythmogenic right ventricular cardiomyopathy. Proc (Bayl Univ Med Cent). 2012;25(4):349.

3. Sugeng L, Moravi V, Weinert L, Niel J, Ebner C, Steringermascherbauer R, et al. Multimodality comparison of quantitative volumetric analysis of the right ventricle. JACC Cardiovasc Imaging. 2010;3(1):10–8.

4. Borgquist R, Haugaa KH, Gilljam T, Bundgaard H, Hansen J, Eschen O, et al. The diagnostic performance of imaging methods in ARVC using the 2010 Task Force criteria. Eur Heart J Cardiovasc Imaging. 2014;15(11):1219–25.

5. Nakajima T, Kimura F, Kajimoto K, Kasanuki H, Hagiwara N. Utility of ECG-gated MDCT to differentiate patients with ARVC/D from patients with ventricular tachyarrhythmias. J Cardiovasc Comput Tomogr. 2013;7(4):223–33.

6. Kimura F, Matsuo Y, Nakajima T, Nishikawa T, Kawamura S, Sannohe S, et al. Myocardial fat at cardiac imaging: how can we differentiate pathologic from physiologic fatty infiltration? Radiographics. 2010;30(6):1587–602.

Aortic Dissection

Xiaohai Ma and Yan Ding

Abstract

Aortic dissection (AD) is the most common entity causing an acute aortic syndrome, generally resulting in the death of the patient. It is defined as the disruption of the medial layer provoked by intramural bleeding, leading to the separation of aortic wall layers and a formation of a true lumen (TL) and a false lumen (FL) with or without communication. In most cases, an intimal tear is an initiating condition, causing the tracking of the blood in a dissection plane within the media [Erbel et al. *Eur Heart J* 35(41):2873–926; 2014]. There are different classifications of aortic dissection. The DeBakey classification includes types I, II, and III. Specifically, type I involves both the descending and ascending aorta; type II only involves the ascending aorta and the arch; type III spares the arch and the ascending aorta [McMahon and Squirrell, *Radiographics* 30(2):445–60; 2010]. The use of the Stanford classification system was recommended by the 2014 European Society of Cardiology (ESC) guidelines. The Stanford type A dissection involves the ascending thoracic aorta and may extend into the descending aorta while the intimal tear in a type B dissection is located distal to the left subclavian artery [Erbel et al. *Eur Heart J* 35(41):2873–926; 2014; Nienaber, *Eur Heart J Cardiovasc Imaging* 14(1):15–23; 2013]. In this chapter, the CT imaging manifestations of the different types of aortic dissection will be discussed based on the following two cases.

30.1 Case of Stanford Type A Dissection

30.1.1 History

- A 43-year-old male had acute chest pain for 30 h.
- He had a 10-year history of hypertension and the highest blood pressure was 160/100 mm Hg.

Physical Examination
- Blood pressure: 120/80 mm Hg; Respiratory rate: 12 time/min
- Heart rate: 80 bpm; without arrhythmia

Electrocardiograph
Standard 12-lead electrocardiograph (ECG) revealed no abnormality.

X. Ma (✉) · Y. Ding
Department of Interventional Diagnosis and Treatment, Beijing Anzhen Hospital, Capital Medical University, Beijing, China

© Springer Nature Singapore Pte Ltd. 2020
Z.-y. Jin et al. (eds.), *Cardiac CT*, https://doi.org/10.1007/978-981-15-5305-9_30

30.1.2 Imaging Examination

The patient had a CT angiography (CTA) of the aorta (Fig. 30.1).

30.1.3 Imaging Findings and Diagnoses

The results of aortic CTA images illustrated that there was an intimal tear at the aortic root and the flap can be observed from the aortic root to bilateral common iliac arteries. The aorta was divided into the true lumen (TL) and false lumen (FL). The TL was compressed and flattened, and the FL was larger than the TL. The coronary artery originated from the TL. The ostium of the left common carotid artery and the right anonymous artery straddled the FL and TL. Besides, an intimal patch was observed in the proximal segment of the left subclavian artery. The opening of the superior mesenteric artery and the celiac trunk straddled the FL and TL. The right renal artery and the left renal artery originated from the FL and TL, respectively. The patient had pericardial effusion and pleural effusion.

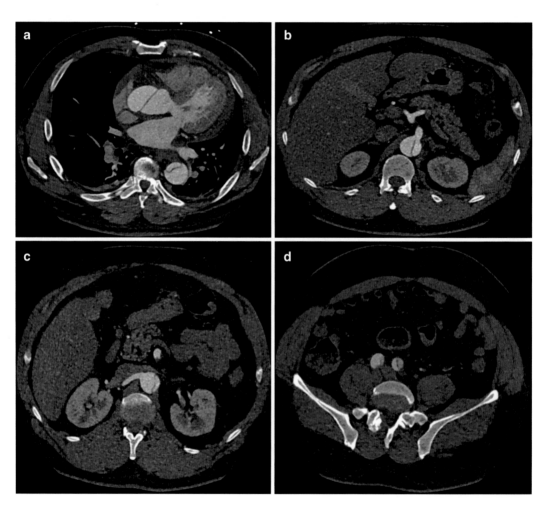

Fig 30.1 CT angiography (CTA) of the aorta, **a-d**: axis CT Images, a: intimal tear at the aortic root; **b**: the celiac trunk originated from TL and FL; **c**: right renal artery originated from FL; **d**: bilateral common iliac arteries involved; **e** and **f**: sagittal and oblique sagittal images; **g**: coronal image; **h**: volume rendering image

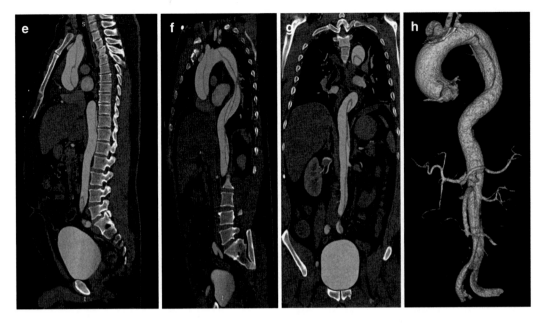

Fig. 30.1 (continued)

30.1.4 Management

This patient underwent an ascending aorta replacement operation.

30.2 Case of Stanford Type B Dissection

30.2.1 History

- A 49-year-old female presented with acute back pain when holding a child, combined with dizziness, headache, nausea, and vomiting.
- She had a 5-year history of hypertension.
- She had an ultrasound of the abdomen in the local hospital and was diagnosed with aortic dissection (Stanford type B).

Physical Examination
- Blood pressure: 153/84 mm Hg; breathing rate: 18 time/min
- Heart rate: 72 bpm without arrhythmia

Laboratory
- D-Dimer: 18,072 ng/ml (elevated)
- Fibrin degradation product (FDP): 183.6 μg/ml (elevated)

Electrocardiograph
Standard 12-lead electrocardiograph (ECG) revealed no abnormality.

30.2.2 Imaging Examination

The patient had a CT angiography (CTA) of the aorta (Fig. 30.2).

30.2.3 Imaging Findings and Diagnoses

Dual-lumen and intima film was observed in the descending aorta, aortic arch, and upper abdominal aorta; there were clots in the FL of the aortic arch to the descending aorta. Besides, the right renal artery was supplied by two branches, and

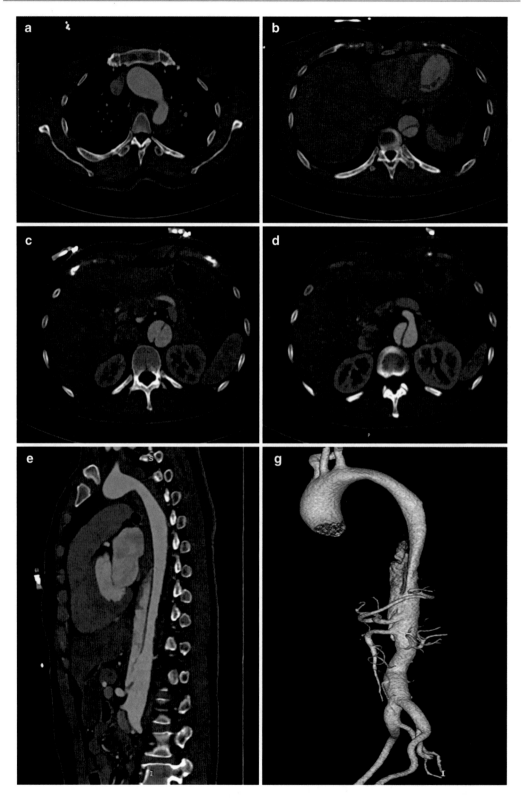

Fig. 30.2 CT angiography (CTA) of the aorta, **a-d**: axis CT Images, show aortic arch, true lumen (TL) and false lumen (FL), intimal tear and the celiac trunk originated from TL separately; **e** and **f**: sagittal and coronal images; g: volume rendering image

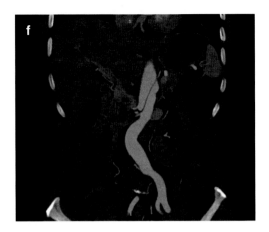

Fig. 30.2 (continued)

the superior branch related to the FL. The superior mesenteric artery, celiac trunk, and left renal artery originated from the TL.

30.2.4 Management

This patient was performed a descending aorta intraluminal stent grafting and Sun's procedure.

30.3 Discussion

AD is a part of the acute aortic syndromes (AAS) that generally has a fatal outcome. It has been reported that the incidence of AD was about six every hundred thousand persons per year in the Oxford Vascular study [1]. Risk factors for aortic dissection are various while the most common one is hypertension that accounts for 60–90% of cases [2]. Cystic aortic wall medical layer necrosis, Marfan syndrome, aortic aneurysm, atherosclerosis,and aortic trauma are also considered risk factors for AD.

The most common symptoms of AD are the abrupt onset of the sharp chest and/or back pain. The pain could be tearing and knife-like that patients almost cannot bear. The most specific characteristic is the sudden appearance. The chest is the most common site of the pain, accounting for 80% of patients. Back and abdominal pain accounts for 40 and 25%, respectively. The pain

can migrate to other sites as AD extends to other areas of the aorta. Clinical presentations and complications also include pulse deficit, aortic regurgitation, myocardial ischemia or infarction [3], heart failure, massive pleural effusions, and end-organ ischemia [2].

The main imaging features of AD on CTA are intimal flap and two lumina. On transverse CT images, flap and dual-lumen can be detected clearly while multiplanar reconstruction (MPR) images contribute greatly to distinguishing and measuring the involvement. Moreover, the precise measurements of the length and diameter of AD, the involvement of aortic branches, and the distance between the intimal tear and the vital branches can be provided by Multidetector CT (MDCT) [4].

Apparently, distinguishing FL and TL is important for endovascular therapy and distinguishing which branch originates from the FL. The diameter of FL is generally larger than that of TL; the flow in the FL is slower; therefore, it may contain thrombus. There may be a slender linear low-density area in FL, representing incompletely dissected media, called the "cobweb sign," which is a specific feature of FL. Besides, the lumen extending to the tail in most cases is the TL.

30.4 Current Technical Status and Applications of CT

Magnetic resonance imaging (MRI) is suitable for diagnosing aortic diseases because it can present the intrinsic contrast between the vessel wall and blood flow. These critical features such as shape, diameter, aorta extent, and the involvement of aortic branches and thrombi can be depicted by MRI. howerver, the use of MRI examination is limited because it is difficult to monitor unstable patients and it takes longer time than CTA [5, 6].

For patients with suspected AD, the protocol of non-enhanced CT followed by CT contrast-enhanced angiography is recommended [7]. CT exhibits an excellent diagnostic accuracy for the detection of AD. Compared with other imaging examinations, the advantages of CT include the complete three-dimensional dataset of the entire aorta, the shorter acquisition and processing time, its widespread practicality [7].

30.5 Key Points

- The main imaging features of AD are intimal flap and two lumina.
- CTA plays a key role in the diagnosis of AD.

References

1. Howard DPJ, Banerjee A, Fairhead JF, Perkins J, Silver LE, Rothwell PM. Population-based study of incidence and outcome of acute aortic dissection and premorbid risk factor control: 10-year results from the oxford vascular study. Circulation. 2013;127(20):2031–7.
2. McMahon MA, Squirrell CA. Multidetector ct of aortic dissection: a pictorial review. Radiographics. 2010;30(2):445–60.
3. Janosi RA, Buck T, Erbel R. Mechanism of coronary malperfusion due to type-a aortic dissection. Herz. 2009;34:478.
4. LePage MA, Quint LE, Sonnad SS, Deeb GM, Williams DM. Aortic dissection: CT features that distinguish true lumen from false lumen. AJR Am J Roentgenol. 2001;177:207–11.
5. Nienaber CA. The role of imaging in acute aortic syndromes. Eur Heart J Cardiovasc Imaging. 2013;14:15–23.
6. Litmanovich D, Bankier AA, Cantin L, Raptopoulos V, Boiselle PM. CT and MRI in diseases of the aorta. AJR Am J Roentgenol. 2009;193:928–40.
7. Erbel R, Aboyans V, Boileau C, Bossone E, Di Bartolomeo R, Eggebrecht H, ESC Committee for Practice Guidelines. 2014 ESC guidelines on the diagnosis and treatment of aortic diseases: document covering acute and chronic aortic diseases of the thoracic and abdominal aorta of the adult. The task force for the diagnosis and treatment of aortic diseases of the European. Eur Heart J. 2014;35(41):2873–92.

Aortic Intramural Hematoma

31

Xiaohai Ma and Yan Ding

Abstract

As a component of the acute aortic syndrome (AAS), aortic intramural hematoma (IMH) is a life-threatening pathologic process that differs from aortic dissection in that it is caused by spontaneous hemorrhage within the media of the aortic wall, without associated intimal rupture or dissection flap. On imaging, the diagnostic criteria are the presence of a circular or crescent-shaped thickening of ≥5 mm of the aortic wall without detectable blood flow [Erbel et al. *Eur Heart J* 35(41):2873–926; 2014]. The extent of IMH can be limited or scattered; besides, the Stanford classification system can also be applied to IMH. The natural progression of IMH is not clear enough yet; its prognosis can be completely absorbed or progressing to aortic rupture, classical dissection, and aneurysm [Von Kodolitsch et al. *Circulation* 107(8):1158–63; 2003]. Accurate diagnosis is of great importance for the management of these patients. Recently, CT especially electrocardiographic gating CT angiogram is the primary technique for the

diagnosis and classification of IMH. In this chapter, the CT imaging manifestations of it will be discussed based on a case of IMH.

31.1 Case of an IMH

31.1.1 History

- A 50-year-old male had severe back pain for 6 h without any alleviation.
- He had a 5-year history of hypertension and the highest blood pressure was 160 mm Hg (systolic pressure).

Physical Examination
- Blood pressure: 140/70 mm Hg; Breathing rate: 14 time/min
- Heart rate: 80 bpm; without arrhythmia

Electrocardiograph
Standard 12-lead electrocardiograph (ECG) revealed no abnormality.

31.1.2 Imaging Examination

CT Images
See Fig. 31.1.

X. Ma (✉) · Y. Ding
Department of Interventional Diagnosis and Treatment, Beijing Anzhen Hospital, Capital Medical University, Beijing, China

© Springer Nature Singapore Pte Ltd. 2020
Z.-y. Jin et al. (eds.), *Cardiac CT*, https://doi.org/10.1007/978-981-15-5305-9_31

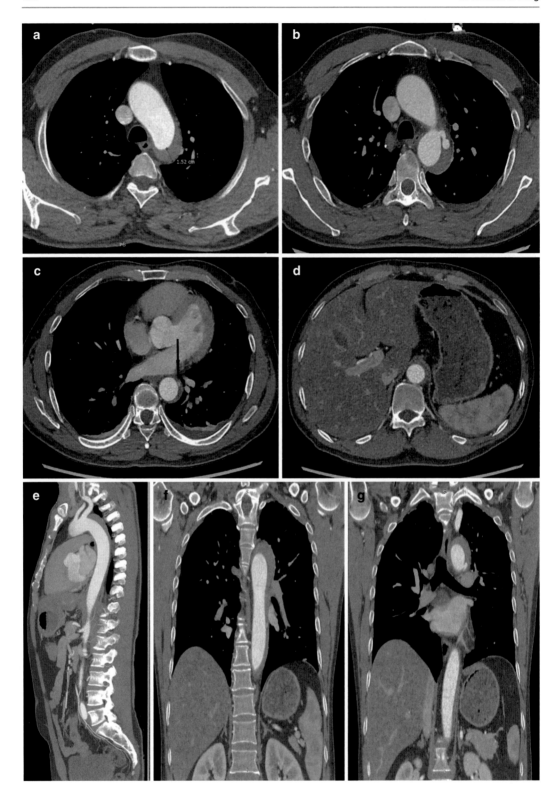

Fig. 31.1 CT angiography (CTA) of the aorta, **a-d**: axis CT Images; **a**: the thickness of the IMH is 15.2 mm; **b**: an ulcer on the aortic arch; **c**: a blood pool in the IMH (black arrow); **d**: IMH extends to the abdominal aorta; **e**: sagittal maximal intensity projection (MIP), indicating low-density hematoma around high-density aorta; **f** and **g**: coronal images exhibit the IMH and the ulcer; **h–j**: volume rendering image

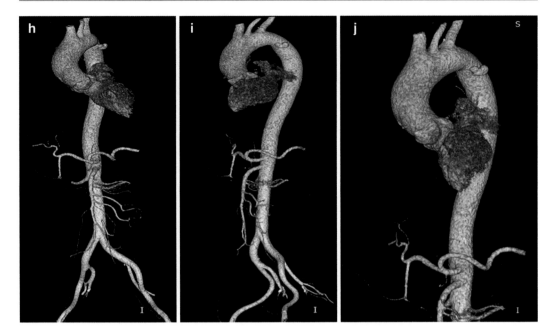

Fig. 31.1 (continued)

31.1.3 Imaging Findings and Diagnosis

The wall of the aortic arch, descending aorta, and upper abdominal aorta was significantly thicker; the thickest part was about 15.2 mm. A niche can be observed in the aortic arch, about 6.3 mm; a hyperdense blood pool in a thoracic aortic hematoma. The wall of the aorta is regular; there is no obvious stenosis or dilation of the lumen, no intimal flap, and double-lumen structure. Bilateral pleural effusion.

31.1.4 Management

- Descending aorta intraluminal stent grafting
- Left common carotid artery-left subclavian artery bypass

31.2 Discussion

IMH accounts for 6% of AAS and the morbidity is higher in Asian cohorts [1]. The etiology of IMH is not clear enough. It may be related to hypertension, aortic atherosclerosis, penetrating atherosclerotic ulcers (PAU), Marfan syndrome, connective tissue disease, congenital aortic valve disease, coarctation of aorta, pregnancy, and so on. The clinical manifestations of IMH are not specific and similar to those of AD. The most common symptoms are chest and/or back tearing pain. Different from AD, the pain of IMH is rarely migratory. Besides, the recurrence of pain is a signal of hematoma deterioration.

There are two classical mechanisms for the formation of IMH. Type 1 is the primary IMH, which is caused by rupture and bleeding of nutrient vessels in the middle of the aortic wall. This is so-called a simple IMH. The aortic intima is smooth and intact, without calcification and atherosclerotic plaque (the case in this chapter is type 1). Type 2 is secondary IMH. There are calcified areas and atherosclerotic plaques on the intima of the aortic wall. The intima could be penetrated by the aortic penetrating ulcer; then, blood enters the middle layer of the aortic wall to form a hematoma. Moreover, some researchers have explored that there may be intimal tears in the early stage of IMH, suggesting that IMH may be an intimal tear with thromboses in the false lumen [1–3].

On unenhanced CT, the aortic wall is crescentic or circular thickening with hyper or slightly hyperdensity relative to the blood pool in the acute phase, which becomes iso-density over time and often exhibits hypodensity in the middle and late stages. This is because fresh bleeding gradually turns into thrombus and organization. A narrow window (width, 200 HU; level, 40 HU) can contribute to detecting lesions on UECT images [1]. The displacement of intimal calcifications is also an essential sign of IMH. CTA is considered to be one of the main methods for aortic diseases. The aortic wall is crescentic or circular thickened without enhancement and obvious hypodensity compared with the hyperattenuating blood pool.

The prognosis of IMH is variable. It may be completely absorbed, partially absorbed or thickened with new ulcerative lesions, absorbed and form an aneurysm, unchanged, thickened with new local hyper-attenuation, classical AD, and aorta rupture. Several imaging factors have been demonstrated to indicate a higher risk for complications or progression, mainly including the location and extent of IMH. Stanford type A IMH results in an increased risk for poor prognoses. IMH with aortic dilatation increases the risk of adverse events. The maximum aortic diameter of Stanford type A IMH exceeds 48–55 mm while type B IMH exceeds 40–41 mm and has a higher risk for adverse outcomes. The thickness of the hematoma is associated with outcomes. The IMH thickness of more than 10–11 mm is at a higher risk for adverse outcomes. Focal contrast enhancement includes two types: the ulcer and the intramural blood pool. An ulcer is a local hyper-attenuation extending from the aortic lumen into the IMH with a visible communication (orifice >3 mm). The intramural blood pool is a similar lesion within the IMH while it has a very small (<2 mm) or imperceptible communication to the aortic lumen. Both two types are risk factors for adverse outcomes [1, 4–6].

31.3   Current Technical Status and Applications of CT

On magnetic resonance imaging (MRI), IMH is characterized by crescentic or circular thickening of the aortic wall. On spin-echo (SE)-T1WI, the thickened wall is of the hyper-intensive signal; on Cine-MR, the hematoma is of the hypo-intensive signal. MRI can distinguish the hematoma phases according to the change of signal on different sequences, which helps evaluate the prognosis. However, it takes a long time for MRI examination and the image quality can be affected by various factors. Echocardiographic evaluation of the aorta is a routine part of the standard echocardiographic examination and it is able to find the intramural hematoma. The thickness of the hematoma and whether there is an intimal flap can be clearly presented by transesophageal echocardiography (TEE), which is of high accuracy in the diagnosis of IMH. Nevertheless, it usually cannot show the entire aorta.

Multislice spiral CT (MSCT) truly realized aortic volume angiography. The acquisition time is shorter, the scanning range is wider and the radiation dose is reduced. Moreover, those imaging factors suggesting poor prognosis in the early stage can also be clearly presented [7]. Dual-source CT can further improve the scanning speed with the coronary artery showed clearly, which is of great value in evaluating the condition of patients [8].

31.4   Key Points

- IMH belongs to AAS without characteristic clinical symptoms and the prognosis is variable.
- Imaging factors play a major role in evaluating the prognosis of IMH.

References

1. Gutschow SE, Walker CM, Martínez-Jiménez S, et al. Emerging concepts in intramural hematoma imaging. Radiographics. 2016;36(3):660–74.

2. Park KH, Lim C, Choi JH, et al. Prevalence of aortic intimal defect in surgically treated acute type A intramural hematoma. Ann Thorac Surg. 2008;86(5):1494–500.

3. Song JK. Aortic intramural hematoma: aspects of pathogenesis 2011. Herz. 2011;36(6):488–97.

4. Evangelista A, Mukherjee D, Mehta RH, O'Gara PT, Fattori R, Cooper JV, et al. Acute intramural hematoma of the aorta: a mystery in evolution. Circulation. 2005;111(8):1063–70.

5. Ganaha F, Miller DC, Sugimoto K, Do YS, Minamiguchi H, Saito H, et al. Prognosis of aortic intramural hematoma with and without penetrating atherosclerotic ulcer: a clinical and radiological analysis. Circulation. 2002;106(3):342–8.

6. Kruse MJ, Johnson PT, Fishman EK, et al. Aortic intramural hematoma: review of high-risk imaging features. J Cardiovasc Comput Tomogr. 2013;7(4):267–72.

7. Kitai T, Kaji S, Yamamuro A, et al. Detection of intimal defect by 64-row multidetector computed tomography in patients with acute aortic intramural hematoma. Circulation. 2011;124(11 Suppl):S174–8.

8. Liang J, Kong L, Jin Z, et al. Initial experience of the application of third-generation dual-source ct scanner in high-pitch angiography of aorta. Zhongguo yi xue ke xue yuan xue bao. Acta Academiae Medicinae Sinicae. 2017;39(1):68–73.

Aortic Aneurysm

32

Xiaohai Ma and Yan Ding

Abstract

Aneurysm is the second most frequent disease of the aorta [Erbel et al. *Eur Heart J* 35(41):2873–926; 2014]. Aneurysm is defined as a limited dilatation of the artery, which is 1.5 times larger than the normal diameter. It is generally divided into the thoracic aortic aneurysm (TAA) and the abdominal aortic aneurysm (AAA) based on the location of the dilatation. Thoracic aortic aneurysms can affect aortic root, ascending aorta, aortic arch, descending aorta, and aortic aneurysms involving the lower thoracoabdominal segment of the diaphragm. An abdominal aortic aneurysm can be divided into the suprarenal abdominal aortic aneurysm, perirenal abdominal aortic aneurysm, and infrarenal abdominal aortic aneurysm according to the distance between the location of the disease and the renal artery. More than 90% of abdominal aortic aneurysms are subrenal type; besides, abdominal aortic aneurysms are more common than thoracic aortic aneurysms. In this chapter, the CT imaging manifestations of the aortic aneurysm will be discussed based on a case of thoracoabdominal aortic aneurysm and a case of an infrarenal abdominal aortic aneurysm.

32.1 Case of TAA

32.1.1 History

- A 57-year-old male had intermittent back pain for 3 months without chest congestion, cardiopalmus, nausea, and vomiting.
- He had a 10-year history of hypertension and 2-year diabetes.

Physical Examination
- Blood pressure: 125/80 mm Hg
- Breathing rate: 20 time/min
- Heart rate: 70 bpm

Electrocardiograph
Standard 12-lead electrocardiograph (ECG) showed ST-T change.

32.1.2 Imaging Examination

CT Images
See Fig. 32.1.

X. Ma (✉) · Y. Ding
Department of Interventional Diagnosis and Treatment, Beijing Anzhen Hospital, Capital Medical University, Beijing, China

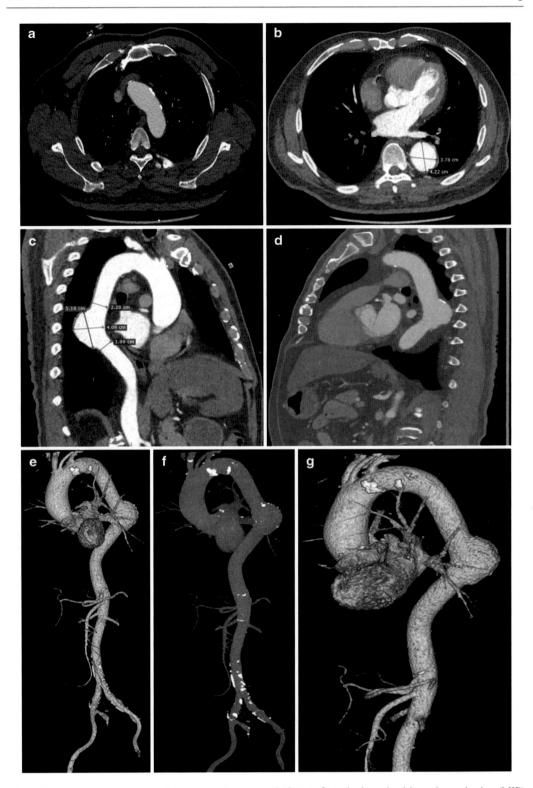

Fig 32.1 CT angiography (CTA) of the aorta. **a-b**: axial CT Images showed calcifications on the aortic arch (the maximum cross-section of the aneurysm is 4.22 × 3.78 cm); **c**: multiplanar reconstruction (MPR) images (the neck of the aneurysm is 2.28 cm, the extent is 5.18 cm); **d**: sagittal maximal intensity projection (MIP) image showed the aneurysm and calcifications on the aneurysm. Volume rendering (VR) (**e, g**) and MIP (**f**) images showed calcifications on the aorta and the aneurysm

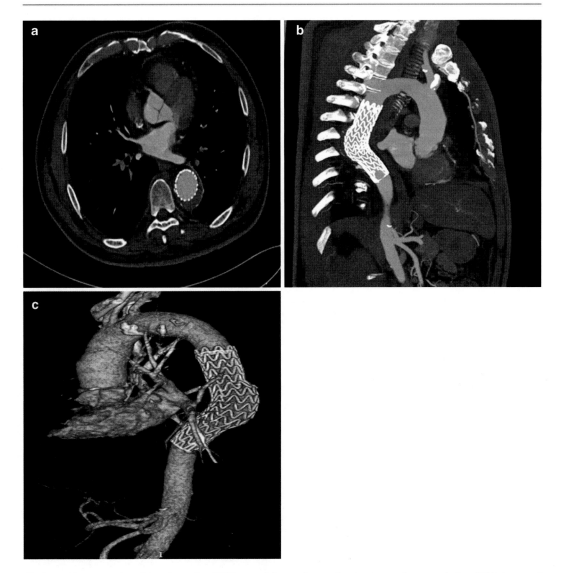

Fig 32.2 Post-operation CT angiography (CTA). **a**: axial CT Image shows the hypo-attenuation thrombosis outside the stent; **b**: MIP image shows the whole picture of the endovascular stent; **c**: volume rendering (VR) image of the aorta and stent

32.1.3 Imaging Findings and Diagnosis

The wall of the aortic arch, descending aorta, and abdominal aorta had irregular incrassation and calcification. The proximal descending aortic lumen dilated. Anteroposterior and vertical diameters of the aneurysm are 4.22 cm and 5.15 cm. Besides, a few hypo-attenuation thrombi were observed in the lumen (Fig. 32.1).

32.1.4 Management

- Thoracic Endovascular Aortic Repair (TEVAR) procedure
- Post-operation aortic CTA (Fig. 32.2)

32.2 Case of AAA

32.2.1 History

- A 67-year-old male has detected an AAA when he received a physical examination 3 days ago.
- He suffered from hypertension while the detail was not clear.

Physical Examination
- Blood pressure: 120/80 mm Hg
- Breathing rate: 12 time/min
- Heart rate: 80 bmp

Electrocardiograph
Standard 12-lead electrocardiograph (ECG) revealed no abnormality.

32.2.2 Imaging Examination

See Fig. 32.3.

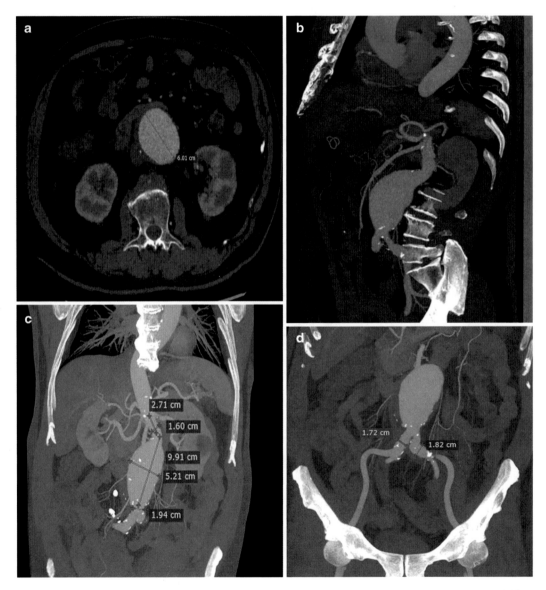

Fig 32.3 CT angiography (CTA) of the aorta. **a**: axis CT Image (the maximum diameter of the aneurysm is 6.01cm); **b–d** and **f**: MIP images (showing the whole aneurysm, bilateral common iliac arteries, and calcifications on the aorta); **e** and **g**: volume rendering (VR) images

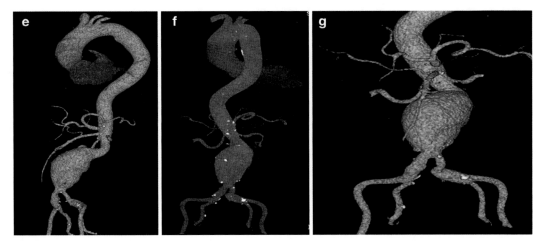

Fig 32.3 (continued)

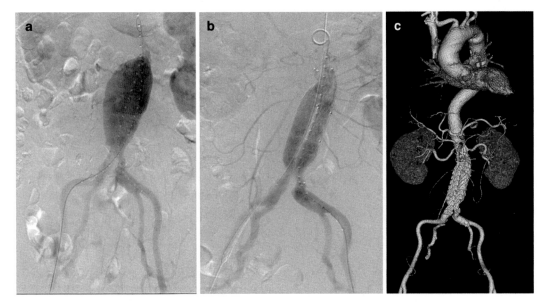

Fig 32.4 Intraoperative digital subtraction angiography (DSA) images (**a** and **b**) show the whole aneurysm and the stent; **c**: postoperative CTA VR image shows the stent and the aorta

32.2.3 Imaging Findings and Diagnoses

The wall of the aortic arch, the descending aorta, and the upper abdominal aorta were irregular; the punctate calcification can be observed. The distal abdominal aorta expanded; the neck is about 1.60 cm; the diameter is about 6.01 cm; the extent is about 9.91 cm. A muscular thrombosis can be observed in the aneu-rysm. The wall of the bilateral common iliac artery and internal iliac artery were irregular and calcified and the lumen of the bilateral common iliac artery was dilated (Fig. 32.3).

32.2.4 Management

- Endovascular Aortic Repair (EVAR) proce-dure (Fig. 32.4)

32.3   Discussion

The etiology of TAA is not clear enough. It may relate to hypertension, aortic atherosclerosis, Marfan syndrome, AD, and trauma. AAA is the result of the interaction of multiple factors such as atherosclerosis, senior, male gender, hypertension, and smoking [1].

Most patients with aortic aneurysms do not have any clinical symptoms and signs; they are often found in physical examinations. Atypical pain is a common symptom and can be a dull pain or swelling pain. Acute pain and shock generally present in the case of a ruptured aneurysm. Compression symptoms occur when AA is compressed into the surrounding organs and tissues. A pulsatile abdominal mass is frequently found in the abdomen of AAA patients.

32.4   Current Technical Status and Applications of CT

Imaging evaluations of AA mainly include: (1) morphological characteristics, true or false aneurysms, cystic or spindle aneurysms; (2) the size and number of AA; (3) the condition of main branches of the aorta (if involved), and the degree of the involvement; (4) the condition of aneurysm lumen, wall, and peritumoral area; (5) etiologies; and (6) complications.

Traditionally, aortography was considered to be the "gold standard" for optimal imaging of morphological characteristics, extent, branches, and the aneurysm lumina. However, the high radiation dose and invasiveness are its disadvantages. The ultrasound is one of the main imaging methods because it can accurately measure the aortic size, detect wall lesions and it is low cost. Recently, CTA and MRI play a major role in the dignosis and the evaluation of the AA. Both of them can present the lesions in multiplane and multiangle, contributing to clarifying the etiology of aneurysms. However, the calcification is clearer on CTA than that on MRI. With the development of CT technology, the temporal and spatial resolution have been better other imaging modalities. Moreover, various post-processing techniques are widely used to evaluate the specific location of the aortic aneurysm, the wall and lumina, and branching vessels. It is of great value for clinicians to decide whether the disease needs intervention and which treatment is suitable. Preoperative evaluations of TEVAR and EVAR include the location, size, shape, wall condition (calcification and/or thrombosis), proximal and distal anchorage areas (length, diameter, and wall condition), branch vessel involvements, surgical approach, etc.

32.5   Key Points

- Most aortic aneurysms require imaging examination for diagnosis.
- CTA is still the most important method for diagnosis and preoperative evaluation.

Reference

1. Golledge J, Muller J, Daugherty A, Norman P. Abdominal aortic aneurysm: pathogenesis and implications for management. Arterioscler Thromb Vasc Biol. 2006;26:2605–13.

Perioperative Imaging of Aortic Root

33

Xiaohai Ma and Yan Ding

Abstract

The common diseases that involve the aortic root and the ascending aorta include aortic valve anatomy and dysfunction, Stanford type A acute aortic syndromes (AAS), including thoracic aortic dissection (TAD), intramural hematoma (IMH), penetrating atherosclerotic ulcer, thoracic aortic aneurysm (TAA), and aortitis [Bhave et al. *JACC Cardiovasc Imaging* 11(6):902–19; 2018]. High-quality imaging of the aorta is indispensable in establishing accurate diagnoses and making optimal treatment plans. In this chapter, the CT imaging manifestations of the aortic root and the ascending aorta will be discussed based on a case of ascending aortic aneurysm with bicuspid aortic valves.

33.1 Case of the Ascending Aortic Aneurysm with Bicuspid Aortic Valves

33.1.1 History

- A 53-year-old male patient without any complaints.

X. Ma (✉) · Y. Ding
Department of Interventional Diagnosis and Treatment, Beijing Anzhen Hospital, Capital Medical University, Beijing, China

- Health examination presented that the diameter of his ascending aorta was 55 mm with bicuspid aortic valves.

Physical Examination
- Blood pressure: 110/80 mm Hg; respiratory rate: 18 time/min
- Heart rate: 80 bpm
- Auscultation: I–II-degree systolic murmur in the aortic area

Electrocardiograph
Standard 12-lead electrocardiograph (ECG) revealed no abnormality.

33.1.2 Imaging Examination

X-Ray
See Fig. 33.1.

CT Images
The patient had aortic CT angiography (Fig. 33.2) and coronary CT angiography (Fig. 33.3).

33.1.3 Imaging Findings and Diagnoses

Chest X-ray image: the ascending aorta dilated and the aortic node broadened (Fig. 33.1). CT images: ascending aortic dilatation combined with bicuspid aortic valves; the maximum diam-

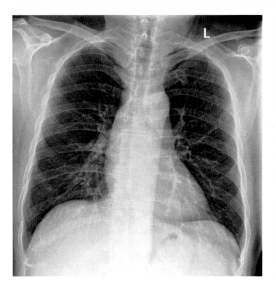

Fig. 33.1 Chest X-ray image: the ascending aorta dilated and the aortic node broadened

eter of the ascending aorta was about 5.32 cm. Calcification can be observed in the aortic root. The coronary CTA presented that coronary arteries originated from two sinuses. The non-calcification plaque in the proximal part of LAD and the lesion were mild stenosis (Figs. 33.2 and 33.3).

33.1.4 Management

- The patient had ascending aorta replacement and aortic valvuloplasty operation.
- The aortic CTA 3 days after the operation (Fig. 33.4) indicated that the diameter of the artificial vessel was 3.03 cm and there were a few hyper-attenuation around the artificial vessel. The pericardial effusion, bilateral pleural effusion, and bilateral atelectasis can be observed.

33.2   Discussion

The aortic root and ascending aorta can be affected by various diseases. Accurate and repeatable aorta measurements are essential to detect and classify aortic diseases and guide treatment decisions. All of these need to be achieved by

imaging examination. The main contents need to be evaluated by imaging before aortic root surgery, including the location and scope of the lesion, the condition of coronary arteries, the aortic root, the heart function, whether there is anatomic variation in the heart, aorta and its branches, etc. Presently, the information mentioned above can mainly be obtained by echocardiography, CTA, and magnetic resonance imaging (MRI); among them, CTA is the most common method.

Two different approaches are employed to aortic CTA: electrocardiographic gating and non-electrocardiographic gating. The electrocardiographic gating should be set to reduce motion artifact because the aorta is a dynamic structure, especially in the aortic root, ascending aorta, and proximal arch [1–5]. Besides, image acquisition should cover the entire cardiac cycle.

The aortic root is an extension of the left ventricular outflow tract. It consists of the sinuses of Valsalva, the fibrous interleaflet triangles, and the valvular cusps themselves. The evaluation of the aortic root and ascending aorta include aortic valve annulus, sinuses of Valsalva, the coronary ostial heights, sino-tubular junction (STJ), coronary arteries and proximal tubular portion of the ascending aorta [3, 6]. An aortic valve annulus is a virtual plane determined by the most basal attachment points of the three aortic valve cusps. The accurate identification and positioning of each three points are the most crucial step that needs standard multiplanar reformats to mark the lowest point of each sinus; besides, the aortic valve annulus plane is automatically generated by measurement software. The average diameter, perimeter, and area could be measured using measurement software. The evaluation of sinuses of Valsalva includes the size, shape, number and location of valve leaflets and the shape and degree of calcification of valve leaflets. The heights of the coronary ostial and STJ should be measured perpendicular to the annular plane. Moreover, MDCT was used to evaluate the position and degree of stenosis of coronary arteries. However, coronary angiography should also be considered to determine the degree of stenosis for patients with severe calcification of coronary arteries.

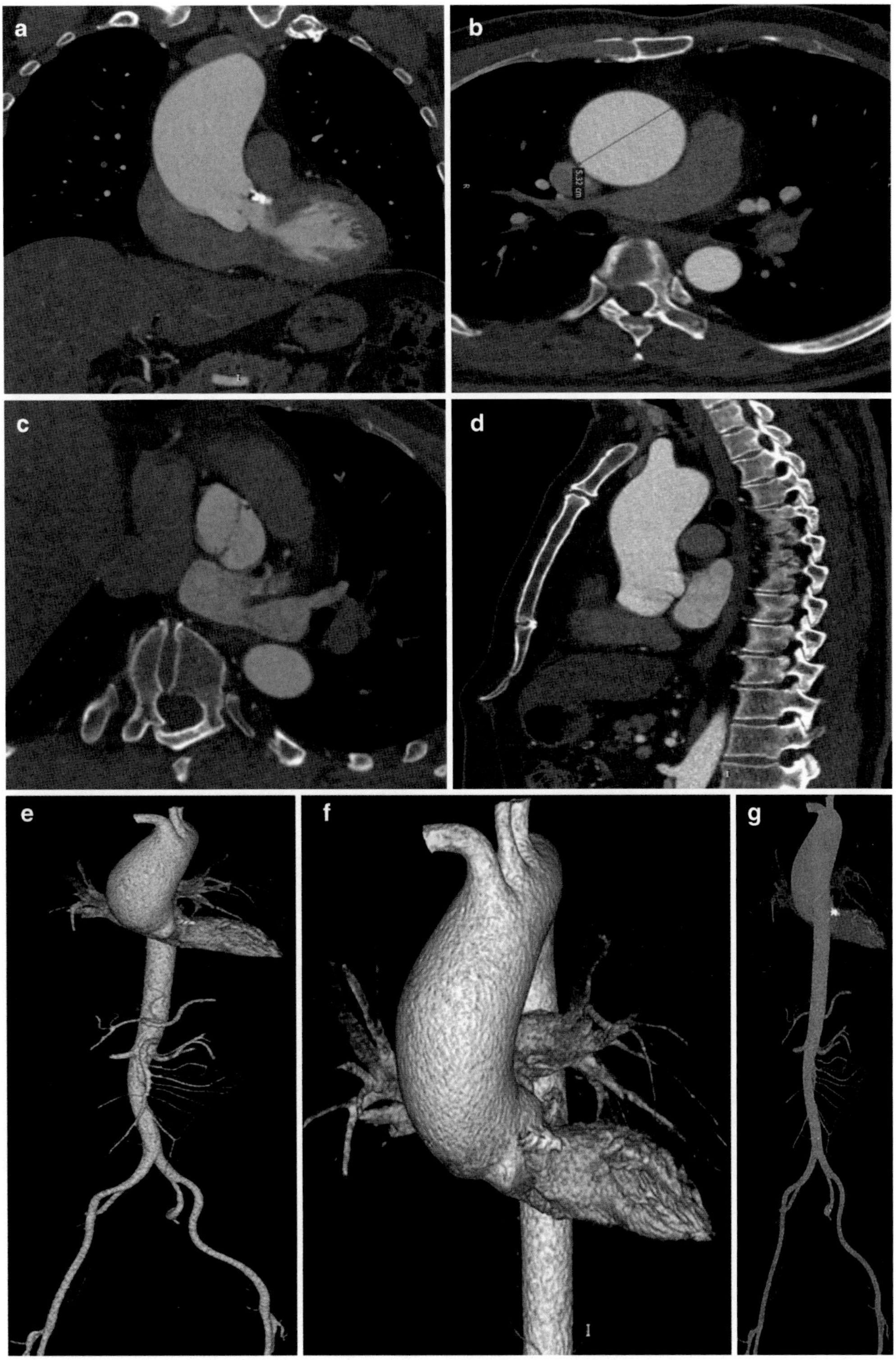

Fig. 33.2 Aortic CT angiography (CTA), (**a**) coronal image showed the calcification of the aortic root and the dilatation of the ascending aorta; (**b**) axis CT image showed that the diameter of the ascending aorta is 5.32 cm; (**c**) oblique axis image showed the bicuspid aortic valves; (**d**) sagittal image showed the dilatation of the ascending aorta; (**e** & **f**) volume rendering images; (**g**) maximal intensity projection (MIP)

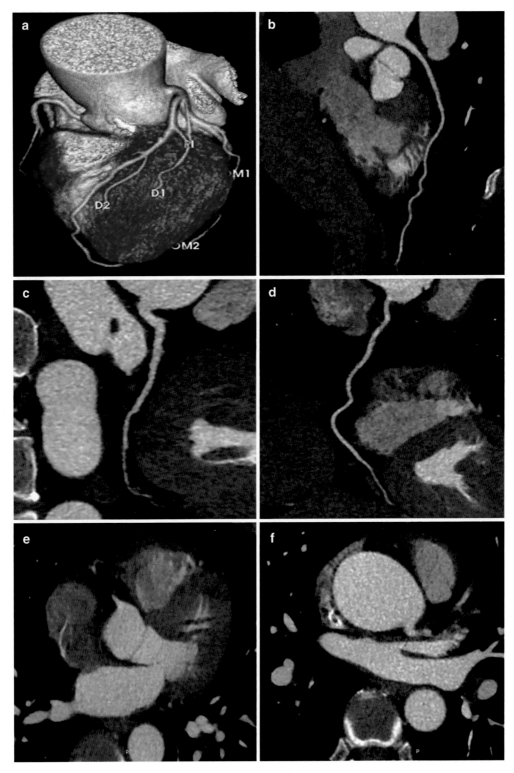

Fig. 33.3 Coronary CT angiography (CTA). (**a**) volume rendering image; (**b** and **c**) curved multiplanar (CPR) reconstructed images; (**b,** left anterior descending [LAD]; **c**, left circumflex artery [LCX]; **d**, right coronary artery [RCA]); (**e** and **f**) axis CT images showed the origins of coronary arteries

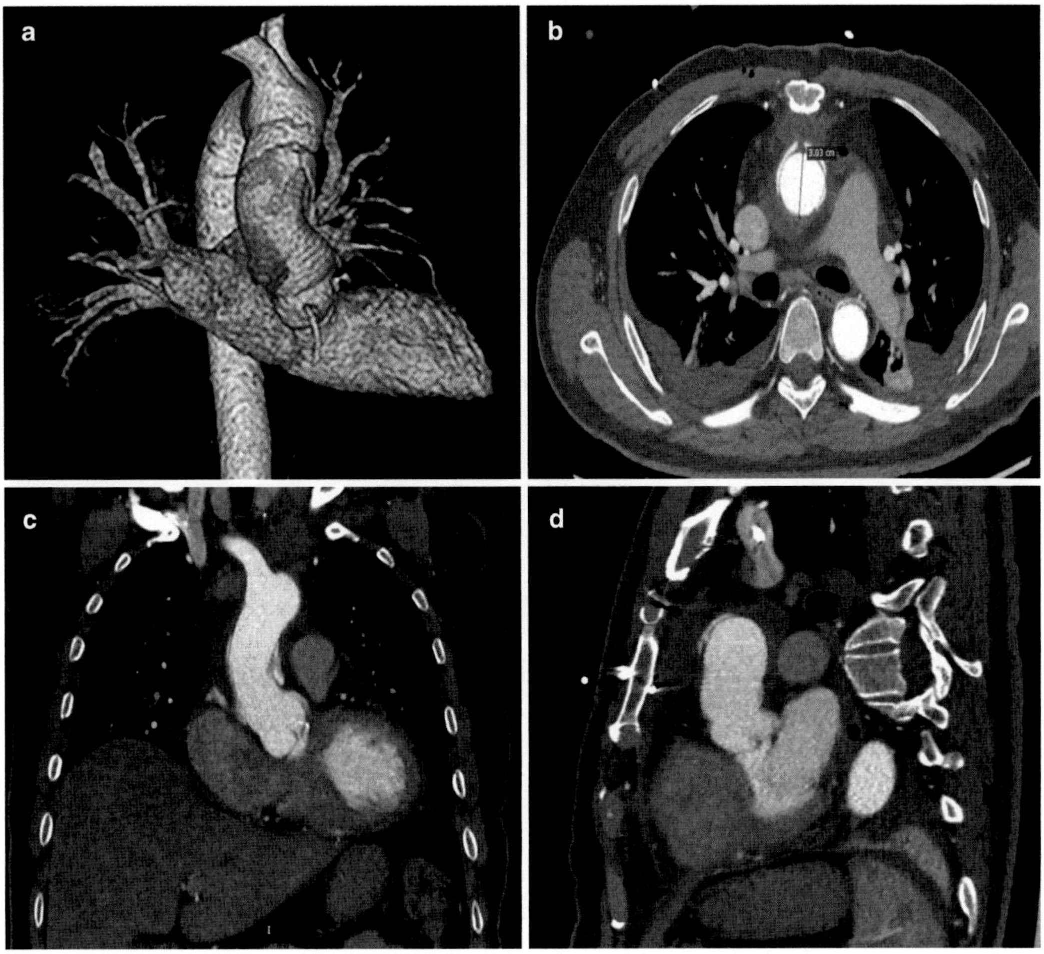

Fig. 33.4 Aortic CT angiography (CTA) after the operation for 3 days. (**a**) the volume rendering image; (**b**) axis CT image showed that the diameter of the ascending aorta is 3.03 cm; (**c** and **d**) coronal image and the oblique sagittal image showed the artificial vessel

After the operation, the aortic CTA must be performed. It is used to evaluate the shape and function of valves and the artificial vessel, the anastomotic condition, whether there is an anastomotic leakage, pericardial effusion and the conditions of surrounding organs such as lungs.

33.3   Current Technical Status and Applications of CT

The echocardiography especially the transesophageal echocardiography (TEE) is widely used in identifying diseases involving the aortic root. However, the image quality of echocardiography is always limited by various factors such as body habitus and the doctors' technical level. Besides, different doctors may have different measurements and assessments for the same patient, resulting in affecting the evaluation of the disease and treatment. At present, the wider applicability of it is limited by the disadvantages of MRI in displaying lesions on multiple planes and contraindications such as a cardiac pacemaker. With the development of CT imaging technology and the postprocessing software, CT has become the central technique. It can accurately measure the parameters of lesions before the operation, display lesions from multiple angles, simulate and generate operative effect pictures, and even combine with 3D printing.

33.4 Key Points

- Aortic CTA plays an essential role in the assessment of preoperative planning and postoperative follow-up of diseases involving the aortic root.

References

1. Bhave NM, Nienaber CA, Clough RE, Eagle KA. Multimodality imaging of thoracic aortic diseases in adults. JACC Cardiovasc Imaging. 2018;11(6):902–19.
2. Hiratzka LF, Bakris GL, Beckman JA, Robert M, Carr VF, Casey DE, et al. Downloaded from content.onlinejacc.org by on March 24, 2010. JAC. 2010;55(14):e27–e129.
3. Blanke P, Weir-McCall JR, Achenbach S, Delgado V, Hausleiter J, Jilaihawi H, et al. Computed tomography imaging in the context of transcatheter aortic valve implantation (TAVI)/transcatheter aortic valve replacement (TAVR): an expert consensus document of the Society of Cardiovascular Computed Tomography. J Cardiovasc Comput Tomogr. 2019;13(1):1–20.
4. Valente T, Rossi G, Lassandro F, Rea G, Marino M, Muto M, et al. Emergency radiology special feature: review article MDCT evaluation of acute aortic syndrome (AAS). (October 2015), 1–19; 2016.
5. Erbel R, Aboyans V, Boileau C, Bossone E, Di Bartolomeo R, Eggebrecht H, et al. 2014 ESC guidelines on the diagnosis and treatment of aortic diseases: document covering acute and chronic aortic diseases of the thoracic and abdominal aorta of the adult. The task force for the diagnosis and treatment of aortic diseases of the European Society of Cardiology. Eur Heart J. 2014;35(41):2873–926. https://doi.org/10.1093/eurheartj/ehu281.
6. Goldstein SA, Evangelista A, Abbara S, Arai A, Asch FM, Badano LP, et al. Multimodality imaging of diseases of the thoracic aorta in adults: from the American society of echocardiography and the European association of cardiovascular imaging: endorsed by the society of cardiovascular computed tomography and society for Cardiovascular Magnetic Resonance. J Am Soc Echocardiogr. 2015;28(2):119–82.